# CELEBRITY ARMS IN A DAY

## Body Sculpting with the New Interactive Lipo Method

# TESTIMONIALS FOR DR. SU'S WORK

*"I found the entire experience to be wonderful. Dr. Su understands how the woman's body is supposed to look and my results surprised even me. I am so happy I had lipo and so happy with Dr. Su. Thank you!"* Abbey from Sarasota

*"They really know how to make you feel confident and comfortable. Thank you to Dr. Su and his awesome team for my new body."*

*"I work in a medical facility, so my expectations are super high. Dr. Su and his staff provided excellent service and quality care. I came to Dr. Su to find my waistline. I seemed to have lost it after my three babies. From my first appointment to my last, I always felt completely at ease. Dr. Su and his staff walked me through every step of my procedure/recovery, and they were there to hold my hand when I needed it! I would definitely recommend Dr. Su's services to friends and family."*

*"This was life-changing for me. I now have more confidence and can enjoy going into a dressing room!"*

*"I am turning 60 soon and wanted to look and feel better about myself. After research and interviewing other doctors for this procedure, I fell in love with Dr. Su and his staff. I couldn't feel better about my decision. The staff is always smiling and so friendly. Dr. Su is so articulate about his work, and takes his time to make it right the first time. My recommendation to anyone will be Artistic Lipo."*

*"Dr. Su IS THE EXPERT in regards to arm sculpting. I am 64 years old, and he was able to greatly improve my "overhang" underarms. He was very realistic with me as to what I could expect. I feel he was able to improve my arms more than I expected possible for my age. I would be happy to speak to potential patients to encourage them to go ahead and have the surgery. Dr. Su IS the artist I read about. Thank you!"*

*"Dr. Su IS truly an artist with liposuction. His consultation was very informative, and he gave me very realistic expectations of the procedure I was interested in. I am older, and despite regular free weight workouts, my upper arms still had "bat wings". When my granddaughter commented on my "jiggling" upper arms, I knew I had to do something! Dr. Su to the rescue!! He showed me how he could considerably improve the sagging and did not promise 100% removal- this would be false expectations. What he did tell me was that he could improve my underarm sagging by 70%. For me, that was realistic and truthful. I am now four months post-op and could not be happier!! My results are more than I expected. My arms no longer shake when I wave and the muscle definition with the fat removed makes me very happy. Other physicians may say they can sculpt your arms, but Dr. Su will do more than simple liposuction. He is a sculptor of the body! Trust no one else!"*

*"As always, I enjoyed seeing the staff. They are great to talk to and are super caring during the procedures. I have been in awe over Dr. Su's work. I recently referred a friend and she was ecstatic over her results, as well as the staff. I wouldn't go to any other doctor for these types of procedures and would travel from abroad just to have him transform my body. Thank you, Dr. Su and Staff."*

*"He is skilled and dedicated at his job, and it shows by the great work he has done on me, as well as the photos I have seen of other patients. I would recommend Artistic Lipo to anyone looking for a better you."*

# CELEBRITY ARMS IN A DAY

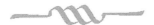

## Body Sculpting with the New Interactive Lipo Method

## DR. THOMAS SU, M.D.

www.artlipo.com

®

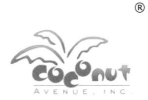

Coconut Avenue ®
Chicago, Illinois USA

The Creative Avenue for Best Selling Authors ®

# Table of Contents

—⁓—

1. Having Arms Like a Celebrity Is Now Possible – In a Day! ............................................. 6

2. Dr. Su's Story: From Artist to Doctor to Artist Again ............................................... 14

3. All Liposuction Is Not the Same ........................................................................... 26

4. Principles of Beauty in Liposculpting .................................................................... 34

5. Dr. Su's New Interactive Lipo Method .................................................................... 44

6. Celebrity Arms: A New Ideal for Women .................................................................. 56

7. The Challenge of Achieving Celebrity Arms .............................................................. 64

8. Creating Celebrity Arms Using Dr. Su's New Interactive Lipo Method ........................ 74

9. Celebrity Arms Gallery ...................................................................................... 86

Glossary of Medical Terms ...................................................................................... 136

Medical Disclaimer ................................................................................................ 139

Model Disclaimer .................................................................................................. 140

Contact Artistic Lipo ............................................................................................. 143

About Coconut Avenue®, Inc. ................................................................................. 145

An Award Winning Publishing Company ................................................................... 146

Other Coconut Avenue® Titles ............................................................................... 147

Other Coconut Avenue® Products ........................................................................... 148

# Chapter 1

Having Arms Like a Celebrity Is Now Possible – In a Day!

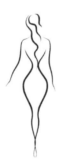

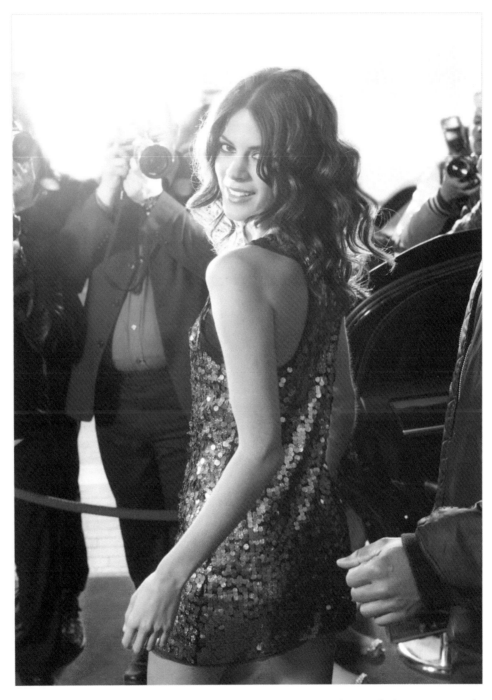

Sculpted arm and shoulder muscles epitomize the Celebrity Arms look.

Aesthetic ideals in our culture are constantly changing. In the past few decades, there has been a shift to a look that embodies fitness. Women today want a shapely, toned body and seek to have more definition in their muscles. In the past, most of the attention women spent on their bodies during fitness routines was focused on their abs, thighs, and buttocks.

Having great-looking, toned arms has become more important in recent years and is now something that women are focusing more attention on. They no longer are satisfied with slimmer arms. Women today want the fit and toned arm look that is being seen and talked about in different celebrity actresses. They want both a shapely and toned look that is now the ideal of arm beauty. Angelina Jolie, Kelly Ripa, and Jennifer Aniston are examples of celebrities who have beautiful arms that epitomize this look.

Many women have tried specific diets or exercise routines to achieve this fit look, with disappointing results. Unfortunately, the arms and shoulders can be one of the most difficult areas of the body to improve, even after spending many hours in the gym. Muscles do get stronger and larger, but this can lead to a bulky look if the fat does not disappear. Diets are also not very effective since they cannot specifically target fat on the arms. Until now, even traditional cosmetic surgery hasn't offered a solution to achieving the toned and fit look that we admire in celebrities.

**The Celebrity Arms look is now possible in just one day!** Dr. Thomas Su,

**BEFORE**

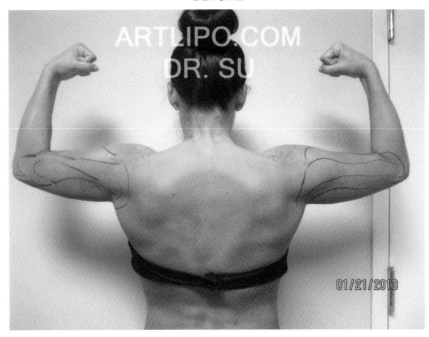

**AFTER**

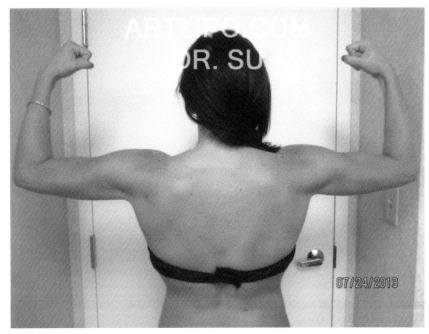

Before and after photographs of a patient who attained the Celebrity Arms look by having the Interactive Lipo Method performed by Dr. Su.

liposuction specialist and surgeon at Artistic Lipo, has developed a revolutionary new method of performing liposuction called the Interactive Lipo Method. This method allows for better liposuction results on all areas of the body. It allows for a very new and exciting way of sculpting the arms that has not been possible until now. Where liposuction of the arm for most surgeons has been restricted to just the lower hang of the arm, the new Interactive Lipo Method allows a surgeon to sculpt the entire arm and shoulder. This results in the defined and toned look that you see in the after photo on the preceding page—a look Dr. Su calls "Celebrity Arms".

You don't have to have great arms to have great results! Women with many different arm types can have great results using this method. Women who work out and are fairly lean can achieve a much more defined and toned look. Also, women who are not particularly active with moderate fat and somewhat looser skin can achieve a very nice toned appearance (see photos on the next page).

Dr. Su's Interactive Lipo Method is done with the patient fully awake using only local anesthesia, which is much safer than when a patient is put to sleep under general anesthesia. The surgery is done in a few hours, and the recovery is very rapid with minimal downtime. The results are visible right away, so patients get to see their results immediately in the mirror before they leave our office. Usually, patients are back to work within a day or two.

**BEFORE**

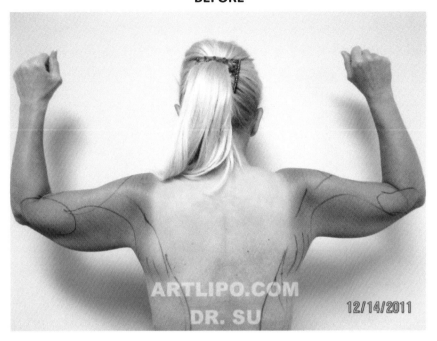

**AFTER**

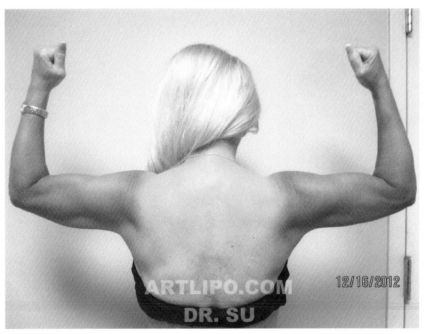

Before and after photographs of another patient with less toned arms
who had the Interactive Lipo Method performed by Dr. Su.

Hopefully, this book will give you a solution to achieving the arms that you've always wanted. The photographs in the Celebrity Arms Gallery presented in Chapter 9 will show you what you can expect, with lots of examples of different arm types. The rest of the book is intended to explain the difficulties of liposuction in general and why the new Interactive Lipo Method is so different and beneficial. The explanation of the concepts in this book is from the perspective of an artist, because Dr. Su has been a lifelong figure artist. Dr. Su's new and unique method is a culmination of years of blending these artistic skills with those of medicine.

# Chapter 2

## Dr. Su's Story:
## From Artist to Doctor to Artist Again

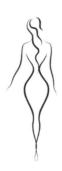

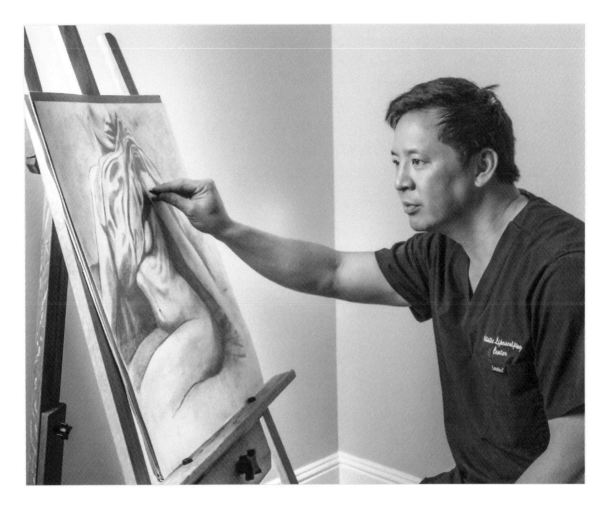

Dr. Thomas Su earned his undergraduate degree in Fine Arts, where he mastered the skills of human figure drawing and sculpting.

My earliest influence in art was watching my mother as a painter. She was a late bloomer, never having any art training or significant experience until she began taking classes in painting when I was quite young. Looking back, I realize that she had always been an artist, but had expressed her artistry in different ways. Our large yard was her canvas, and she had the greenest thumb in the neighborhood—she won the Yard of the Month award many times from the local garden club. She also won many flower arranging competitions. When she began painting, it was in watercolors, and she rapidly advanced to oil paints. In a few short years, my mother was an accomplished painter who was able to re-create the masterpieces of many famous artists. She was able to duplicate Monet's *Water Lilies* perfectly, as well as other masters' paintings of still lifes and flowers. I definitely inherited some of these artistic genes.

My interest in art began near the age of ten after watching her create those beautiful works and wanting to emulate her. My subject matter was totally different, however. I was into monsters, adventure heroes, and wildlife. I started off with pen and pencil. To this day, I continue to love drawing, and still find charcoal and pencil to be my favorite mediums. As I entered my teenage years, I became enthralled with girls and the female form. I learned to draw sexy heroines as well as heroes. I took pride in drawing faces as well and found that girls enjoyed posing for me to do their portraits. An artist must have a muse.

As luck would have it, I was accepted to a magnet high school—Louisiana School for Math, Science, and the Arts. Although I was a math and science

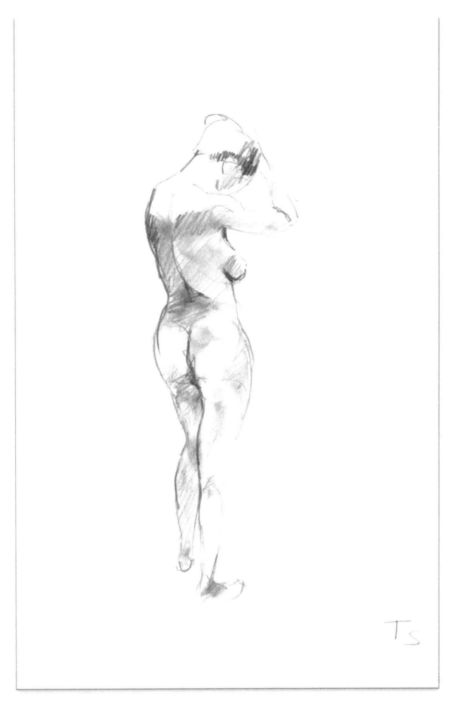

Live nude sketch created during college by Dr. Thomas Su.

guy, this school had some of the finest art teachers in the area, and I was able to take college-level art classes to satisfy my passion. I learned quite a lot in painting and drawing classes. During this period, I competed in interschool art competitions and won several awards. I was very proud to win the Best of Show Award in the school art contest as well. This honor was quite unexpected, as the entry was a quick watercolor portrait of my roommate and was one of the first watercolor paintings I had done.

Entering into college at Rice University, I was influenced by my father to go into engineering, as this was his profession. My first two years were filled with math and science courses. My electives, however, were all art courses. Most of all, I was fascinated to take Life Drawing. I was especially thrilled because I not only got to draw from live models, but it was the first time I had drawn the nude figure. By the end of my sophomore year, I had taken several more Life Drawing figure classes and a couple of courses in sculpting.

Then, a life-changing event happened. As someone who had always made A's and B's, I was actually failing thermodynamics—one of the core subjects on my way to becoming an engineer. This failure made me realize that I did not truly want to become an engineer. I made the decision to change from engineering and to pursue a career in medicine. Specifically, I could see myself becoming a plastic surgeon, combining my love of art and the human figure with a medical career. It wasn't difficult to adjust my major. There were only a smattering of prerequisites for medical school that I still needed, and I decided to double major in both biology and art.

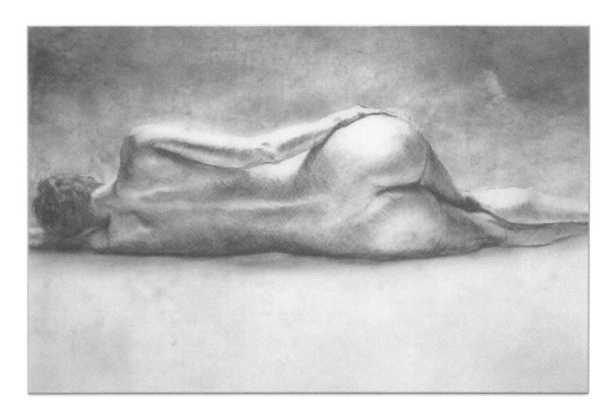

Drawing of a nude figure by Dr. Thomas Su.

I continued to take hands-on art courses where I could explore art of the human figure including lithography, sculpting, and painting. I also had a significant exposure to art history.

By the end of my senior year at Rice University, I had completed the coursework for my Bachelor of Fine Arts degree. At that point, I had been accepted into medical school, so I decided to enjoy my senior year instead of pushing myself to finish the biology major as well. I came three hours short of achieving the biology degree. I wasn't disappointed that I didn't finish the biology degree, but it was much to my father's chagrin. He was a bit disappointed that I only achieved a Bachelor of Fine Arts and not a Bachelor of Science. To me, being accepted into medical school with an Arts degree was a matter of pride. To this day, I have never met another doctor with Fine Arts as their college major.

Medical school at the University of Texas at San Antonio was an amazing time, but four years and a lot of challenging new experiences can change the best of plans. I never lost my love of art. In fact, I designed several class T-shirts featuring artwork of the human figure, which sold out completely. My experiences while on surgery rotations, however, soured my dreams of becoming a plastic surgeon. While I did well on those rotations, my impression of the surgery residents and attending physicians was very disappointing. It seemed to me that there was an overall cutthroat and demeaning attitude, which I felt I could not tolerate for the next seven years. At the time, my experience working in internal medicine seemed to be more rewarding and a better fit for my personality. Thus, I became a

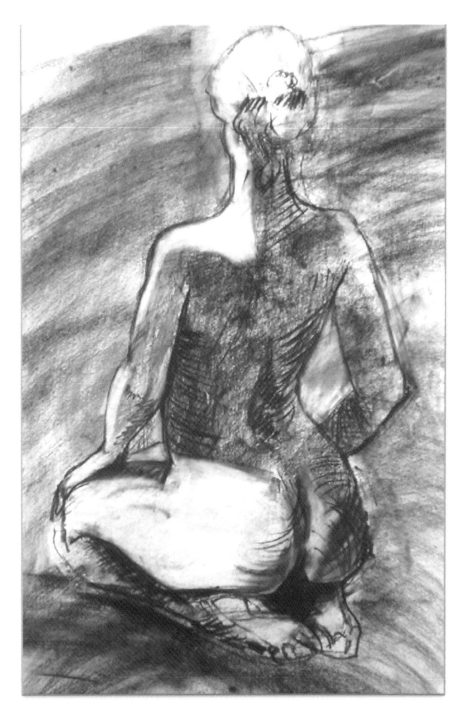

Live nude sketch from college by Dr. Thomas Su.

specialist in Internal Medicine. I became an intellectual "Doctor's Doctor"—knowing and treating disorders of every kind, and understanding all aspects of every organ system. My passion for art now had no place in my career and took a back seat for eight years during my practice in internal medicine. Although I was a very good internist and enjoyed many aspects of it, I felt that there was something missing. Feeling the need to do something creative, I quit internal medicine. I left my practice thinking I might go back to school in architecture, where at least I would be able to create and be artistic. Years earlier, I had gone from being an artist to being a doctor. Now, I was about to go from being a doctor to being an artist once again.

When I left my internal medicine practice, I knew I would never go back, but I didn't have a definite idea of what I was going to do next. The trend of medical spas was just beginning to grow in popularity. This seemed like an avenue where I could exercise my artistic abilities and still be a physician. It took six months from the time I began taking courses to do non-invasive cosmetic procedures until I was able to open my med spa, Radiance Clinique. I offered the standard fare of Botox®, fillers, chemical peels, photo rejuvenation, laser hair removal, and cellulite therapy. I quickly became very good at injectable therapy, and got constant feedback that my patients were very happy. I really enjoyed the injectables since I was able to use my artistic skills to influence the results. With laser and light treatments, however, the results seemed to depend primarily upon technology. At that point, I was ready to find something more challenging for myself, especially from an artistic standpoint.

In 2007, I was introduced to the concept of awake liposuction using local anesthetic. When I first heard about this, I had my doubts. But, after

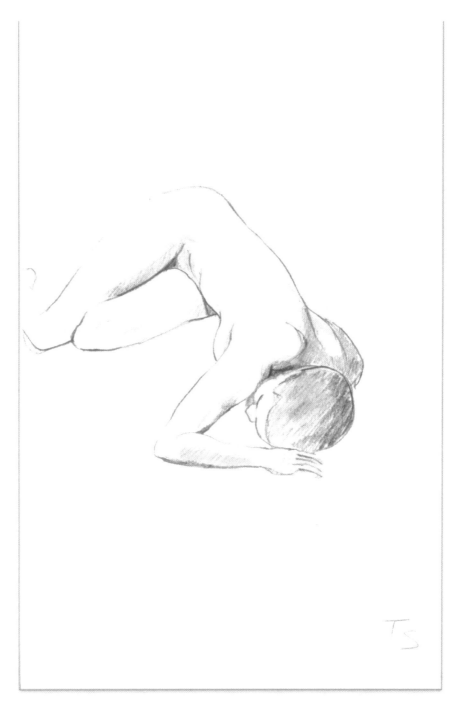

Live nude sketch from college by Dr. Thomas Su.

research into the history of liposuction, I found that this technique had been around for more than twenty years, and there were many studies proving its safety compared to traditional liposuction under general anesthesia. I enrolled in a course and found myself learning liposuction under the instruction of Dr. Dwight C. Reynolds, a liposuction surgeon who had trained hundreds of other physicians in the use of liposuction, VASERlipo®, and SmartLipo™. While I felt very comfortable and natural performing the procedure, I could tell that this was something different and awkward for some of the other students in the class. It was very encouraging to me that at the end of the class, Dr. Reynolds praised me as the best student. I returned from liposuction training ready to get started, but I had no idea that I was about to embark on my new career path.

From the first month that I offered liposuction at my med spa, I became too busy doing liposuction to spend time doing any other procedure. I hired a nurse practitioner to perform all other services, and I did liposuction exclusively on a full-time basis. About a year later, I decided to change the name of the practice to Artistic Lipo. I felt this was an appropriate name since I truly believe that great results are created only when you blend artistic skills with the liposuction. I had finally found a career where I was truly happy. I was doing something that I loved, that was challenging, and that I was good at.

Being both a perfectionist and an artist has always caused me to be my own worst critic. Even at the beginning of my career, I was creating better liposculpting results than the average surgeon and many of my patients were happy. Still, there were many times that I wished I could do better. I wanted to sculpt smoother and I wanted more complete results. I was constantly critiquing my own work and looking for ways to make my results better.

To improve my skills, I initially did what any other professional would do. I joined several cosmetic surgery societies and began attending conferences where I could listen to experts lecture on liposuction. I subscribed to journals on cosmetic surgery and bought all the books I could find pertaining to liposuction. I attended live workshops offered by other surgeons in the field. I found that the information I was hearing was mostly basic and repetitive. I came to a point where I had heard enough about topics such as "complications," "what to watch out for," and "what not to do." What was surprising to me was that the answers to the questions that were the most important to me—"How can I sculpt more smoothly?" and "How can I sculpt more completely?"—were the ones that I couldn't find.

Consequently, my development as a liposuction specialist who was striving to achieve the most beautiful results has largely been self-taught. To my great benefit, having a background as a figure artist provided a wonderful foundation for me to fall back on. Compared to most cosmetic surgeons who have never taken an art course on the human figure, I had many years of experience. What I developed over the past eight years as my own unique method was something that evolved naturally, incorporating different artistic principles and techniques. At this point in my career, I am no longer a novice and am glad to be introducing a revolutionary method that can benefit all surgeons. It is the future and the possibilities for further improvements in liposculpting, however, that keeps this exciting for me.

# Chapter 3

—•—

# All Liposuction Is Not the Same

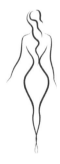

Contrary to what many people think, all liposuction is not the same. Obtaining good liposuction results is not as straightforward as it might seem. There can be vast differences in the outcomes from one surgeon compared to another. It is not as easy as finding a board certified surgeon who will do the surgery for the right price. It is also not about finding the surgeon with the latest equipment or technology. If you have already done research into liposuction, it may have been confusing to read about all the different types—including SmartLipo™, VASERlipo®, and Aqualipo®, just to mention a few. When it comes to liposuction, a lot of hype surrounds new technologies as they are brought to the marketplace. Most of this hype is marketing gimmicks. All types of liposuction eventually rely on a cannula to sculpt and remove the fat. Regardless of the actual instrumentation being used, therefore, the most important factor that determines a patient's outcome or results is a surgeon's skill and experience.

Liposuction is an artistic process, with the aesthetics of the result dependent mainly on the surgeon's abilities. Many people assume that the outcome will be good as long as a surgeon is well-credentialed. Even with a degree from the best university and training hospital, however, a surgeon may not necessarily be the best at liposuction. Even though a plastic surgeon may have a great reputation for doing breast augmentation or face lifts, he or she may not perform good liposuction. Sculpting the fat layer on the body is one of the most difficult surgeries to master, and many plastic surgeons never do enough liposuction in their practices to become skilled at it.

Using abdominal liposuction as an example, the results can differ tremendously from surgeon to surgeon. One surgeon might do a moderate

**BEFORE**    **AFTER**

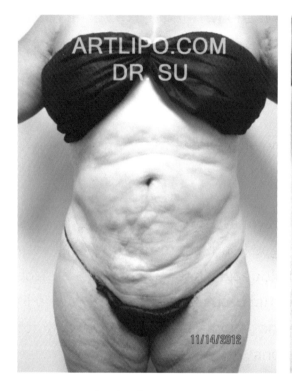 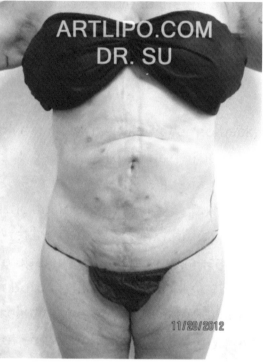

The before photograph shows an example of poorly done
abdominal liposuction. The same patient is shown after
liposuction correction was performed by Dr. Su using
the Interactive Lipo Method.

removal of half of the fat resulting in a smaller appearance, but with noticeable fat remaining. In contrast, another surgeon might remove the fat more completely resulting in a completely flat abdomen. Of course, most patients expect completeness. Completeness takes more time and skill. For a full explanation of completeness, which is one of the principles of beauty relating to liposuction, see Chapter 4.

Problems arise when a surgeon is not skilled at taking fat smoothly, which can lead to a very lumpy and uneven shape (see the example on the previous page). Other major problems occur when a surgeon is not skilled at identifying the best shape for the patient and cannot even visualize the best curves to be sculpted. Another challenge is that bulges and hangs take special skills and experience to master. There are big differences in results if these things are handled skillfully or not. Finally, when performing a specific area of sculpting, the result has to be blended smoothly into surrounding areas. This can be challenging at times even for an experienced surgeon and appears as a noticeable mismatch when not done properly.

In talking to patients, one of the most common misconceptions is that liposuction is about "suctioning out" fat. This would imply that fat is a soft or fluid substance that can be easily vacuumed up. It would also imply that fat can move about freely and smooth itself out if not removed smoothly to begin with. If fat actually flowed in this manner, it would be possible to stick a suction device into the fat layer in one spot and remove it all. This does not happen, however, and fat does not smooth itself out.

Understanding the fat layer on a basic level can help explain why surgeons have difficulty creating a beautiful shape every time. Fat is actually a soft substance, but it is held together by millions of strands of connective fibers. The fibers act like the roots of a plant in soil by holding everything together. When a surgeon is performing liposuction, he or she must break the fat globs away from the fibers.

The instrument a surgeon uses to remove the fat is called a cannula, which is a thin metal tube connected to a handle. The tube is similar in size and shape to a thin straw and has holes on it sides close to the tip. The instrument acts similar to a file, and the holes at the end are like the ridges of a file. This simple instrument is connected to a soft, flexible plastic tube which provides the suction pressure. The cannula is used internally to scrape fat and to break it free from the connective fibers. The suction tube then carries the fat globs away into a canister.

Therefore, liposuction is actually more like sculpting than suctioning. The cannula can be compared to an artist's file, rasp, or chisel in its action. Just as a sculptor takes a little bit of material with each stroke of their tool, so does the liposuction surgeon. The word "liposculpting," which is used throughout this book, is just a more accurate and artistic term than liposuction. A sculptor who works on wood must be precise when he removes the excess material. The liposuction surgeon working on fat must do the same. In this regard, the skills required for artist and surgeon are quite similar.

Because of the connective fibers holding the fat layer together, the fat can be very difficult to remove. Sometimes the fat is soft and comes out easily, but other times the fat can be very fibrous and very difficult to control.

Trying to move through this fibrous fat smoothly and evenly is the challenge, because it will continuously try to bunch up. This is why a surgeon may have a very difficult time removing fat smoothly. Unless the fat is removed smoothly in the first place, the result will not be smooth in the end.

Another factor affecting the beauty of the results is the smoothness and shape of the overlying layer of skin. Everyone wants their skin to be smooth after liposuction, but unless the fat is removed skillfully, an irregular surface or unwanted folds and creases may result. Knowing whether to sculpt closer to the skin or deeper in the fat layer can also make a big difference in how the skin behaves in the end. It takes a tremendous amount of skill and experience to know how to handle looser skin types and create consistently smooth results for these patients.

Finally, there is an even bigger challenge for the liposuction surgeon as compared to a sculptor. Although liposuction is about sculpting on fat, it behaves differently than any other material a sculptor works on. An artist sculpting on wood has a stable form to work on. However, the liposuction surgeon must sculpt a shape that changes with body positioning, as the shape is affected by gravity. When a patient is standing, a bulge on the belly may be quite prominent, but when the patient lies down the bulge disappears. How is a sculptor supposed to shape something he or she cannot see? This issue will be discussed in Chapter 5.

Hopefully, this explains why well-trained and experienced cosmetic surgeons still have difficulty producing consistently beautiful results for all their patients. All of the factors described above contribute to why liposuction is so difficult and why so few surgeons master this art. Many surgeons are good at reducing the bulk of the fat and making an area smaller. Beautiful results, however, are not about just removing fat. An artistic approach and following general principles of beauty are required.

ALL LIPOSUCTION IS NOT THE SAME

# Chapter 4

—ɯɯ—

# Principles of Beauty in Liposculpting

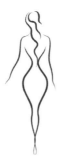

When defining beauty of the human figure, there are aesthetic principles that apply. Some of these principles are universal for most cultures, and some vary according to cultural preferences or current trends. Even if we don't understand these principles of beauty, all of us are capable of identifying a beautiful figure or face when we see one. In fact, as human beings, we are captivated by beauty and will often spend more time looking at someone who is considered beautiful than someone who is not. The ability to identify human beauty is innate in all of us.

What is not common or natural to all people, however, is the ability to look at an object that is not beautiful and realize exactly what it needs to become beautiful. This is the job of a specialist who has a trained eye. For example, consider a run-down house with old carpet and peeling paint. Many people are unable to imagine the true potential a house like this could have. A skillful interior designer, however, would be able to create a beautiful renovation of this house in their mind and make it become reality. Another example is a master hair stylist, who is able to visualize the perfect hair style for their client before actually creating it. You may have heard the quote by the famous artist Michelangelo describing his sculpture, "I saw an angel in the stone and carved until I set it free." This ability to visualize the potential for beauty is the most important trait a liposuction surgeon can possess. Without it, a beautiful result will never be possible.

If we take the human form or shape and look at it from an artistic standpoint, we can identify a number of different features that make it look more or less beautiful. Through liposculpting, a surgeon removes fat and shapes a patient's body by making carefully selected areas smaller, while

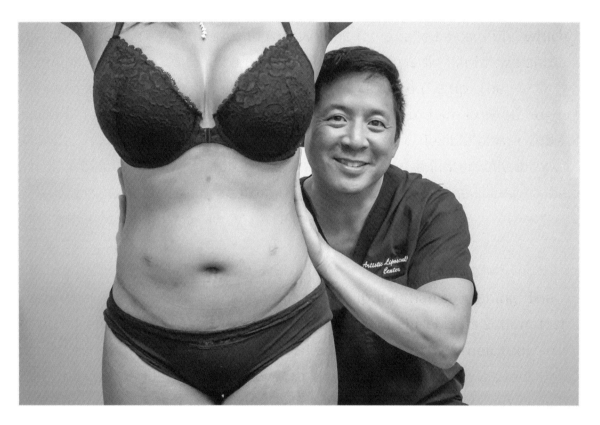

Visualizing a patient's shape in front of a mirror is an important step for the doctor as well as the patient. Here, Dr. Su is holding in the fat on the waist to show his patient what the final result will look like.

leaving other areas alone. For a surgeon to achieve the most beautiful shape in a body, certain principles have to be followed in the liposuction process. When a surgeon achieves these principles, a patient will look the best for their particular body. These principles of beauty for the surgeon are completeness; smoothness and blending; and shape and proportion.

## ❖ Completeness

Although it may seem obvious that the principle of completeness is very important in liposuction, it is not necessarily a common thing that is seen in practice. Certainly, the more completely the fat layer is removed, the more noticeable the result will be. Likely, the patient will be happier with this result. What is seen with liposuction surgeons, however, is that many will do only a fifty to sixty percent removal. Some surgeons do even less. It is less common for a liposuction surgeon to remove fat completely in the eighty to ninety percent range.

Reasons for the differences among surgeons vary. Throughout their training, many surgeons are taught to avoid sculpting into the layer of fat that lies just below the skin. The reasoning behind this is that irregularities are more visible when they closer to the skin. Therefore, leaving a thicker layer of fat just below the skin will keep the results smoother. Unfortunately, some surgeons just don't want to take the time to remove fat more completely. It takes more than double the time to take ninety

BEFORE                                      AFTER

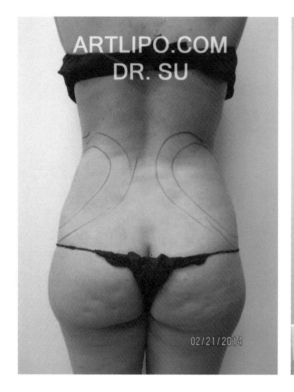
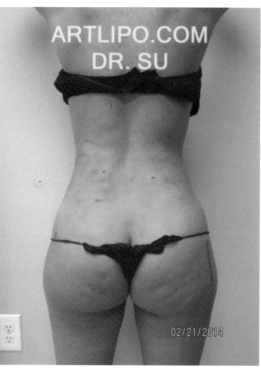

The before photo is a patient who had liposuction of her waist performed incompletely by another surgeon. The after picture shows a nice improvement after the remaining fat was removed by Dr. Su. Her curve was slightly outward before and became slightly inward after her second procedure. Notice how this also makes a nice improvement in her bottom.

percent of the fat layer as opposed to just fifty percent. This is because the technical difficulty increases when fat is removed closer to the skin. It also takes a lot of extra skill for a surgeon to remove fat more completely and keep the skin smooth. The example shown on the preceding page illustrates the principle of completeness. The before picture shows a patient who had already undergone liposuction of her waist by another surgeon. She was disappointed because she could still grab a significant layer of fat after her initial surgery. She had a second surgery of her waist done by Dr. Su, who was able to remove enough additional fat to create a noticeable improvement in her results.

## ❖ Smoothness and Blending

Smoothness and blending are equally important principles in liposuction. A patient could have their fat removed very completely from an area, but if the result is not smooth or well-blended, the patient will likely be disappointed. Most patients would rather have a smooth bulge than have an area that is flatter but looks uneven or rippled.

The smoothness of an area refers to the surface contour of the area being worked on. It is imperative for the liposuction surgeon to remove the fat in a smooth and even fashion, which is not easy. If the skin is looser on a patient, the fat layer attached to it will be much more difficult to control during the surgery, which can lead to irregularities. Certain irregularities are not visible at all until a patient is upright, where gravity comes into play. These irregularities could appear as waviness, unevenness, or creases.

Blending refers to the edges of an area that is being worked on. Most of the areas being treated in liposuction can be described as fat pads. A fat pad is often oval in shape and stands out from the surrounding body area. An example of a fat pad is the outer thigh bulge. If an area is well-blended, the borders of the area being sculpted will mesh seamlessly with its surroundings. If an area is not well-blended, there may be a remnant of the bulge that may look like a rounded ridge. Poor blending can also appear like an indentation or a sharp edge. As with other irregularities that are accentuated by gravity, the lower edge of an area can often form a bulge when a person stands up. These bulges are imperceptible when a patient is lying on the table. Performing good blending, therefore, is a difficult skill to master and takes lots of practice.

## ❖ Shape and Proportion

Creating beautiful shapes in the body is what liposculpting is all about. Finding the most beautiful shape, however, can be difficult for both patients and for novice liposuction surgeons. Shape and proportion refer to looking at a patient from a broader scope and not just at the area being treated. It is important to consider how shaping one area of the body will affect the other areas around it. It is also important to keep in mind that the overall shapes we are trying to create may vary, and include inward curves, outward curves, and straight lines. Creating proper shapes that flow smoothly from one area to another is critical.

Cosmetic surgeons often like to talk about the concept of proportions. This refers to size of one area in relation to another. For instance, the female bust-waist-hip proportion of thirty-six, twenty-four, thirty-six has long been thought to be the most beautiful. Rather than focus on one ideal, however, it is more valuable to discuss this principle in general.

Many patients coming in for evaluation are confused about what areas they should have sculpted to look their best. Often, I have patients requesting arms, abdomen, waist, and thighs—all on their initial consult. Although we could probably do all of these areas on this patient, it may not be practical from a cost standpoint. I can often show a patient what areas will make the most impact without doing every area.

For example, the abdomen and waist are areas that, when sculpted properly, will leave a flat abdomen and a curved-in waistline. When corrected to a smooth "hourglass" shape, the waistline can transform the appearance of the buttocks, thighs, arms, and breasts. This happens because the proportions have been improved and because we create a flowing inner curve (the waist) transitioning into a flowing outer curve (the hip and outer thigh). This principle is shown in the illustration on the next page.

Another example is that a female leg should be narrowing and tapering from the upper thigh down to the knees. The knee should be narrower than the upper thigh. Sometimes, a surgeon will remove fat from the inner thigh but will ignore the bulge at the inner knee. The proportions then become skewed and the leg does not look its best. The upper leg can then look like a log, with the same thickness from top to bottom.

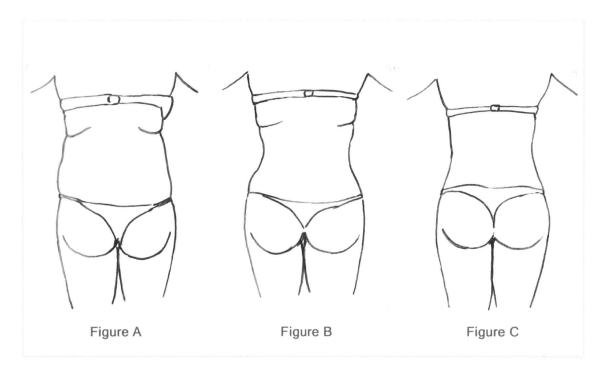

Figure A          Figure B          Figure C

Sketch by Dr. Su illustrating possible liposuction results. Figure A represents the appearance before liposuction. Figure B shows the results of poorly done liposuction—with bumps and waviness. Figure C shows an hourglass figure that is achieved through skillful liposculpting—with more completeness, blending, and a better shape and proportions.

Each area of the body has its own specific shape and curves. That is why a surgeon must be both skilled artistically and experienced enough to recognize these principles. It is not always enough to listen to what a patient says they want. It is important to discuss options with a patient and show them how sculpting one area may affect another. A good surgeon will also explain why it may be important to work on additional areas to create a complete flowing curve or shape. In the illustration on the preceding page, Figure B shows a patient who only had her waist sculpted, which is what patients often request. This liposuction lacks completeness, which resulted in bumps and waviness where the liposuction was not properly blended. Figure C, however, shows the same patient where the waist, hips, and mid-back were sculpted to create a complete hourglass figure and resulting rounded bottom. This resulted in a shape and proportion that is complete, smooth, and aesthetically pleasing.

# Chapter 5

## Dr. Su's New Interactive Lipo Method

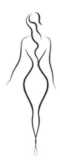

## ❖ Improving on Awake Liposuction

Awake liposuction, which is done using local anesthetic only, is a very popular procedure. Preference for having liposuction done awake is increasing and may have already surpassed the traditional method of placing patients under general anesthesia. Developed in 1986 by Dr. Jeffrey Klein, awake liposuction is also known as tumescent liposuction. Using only local anesthetic is much safer than putting a patient asleep under general anesthesia and is well tolerated by most patients. Apart from safety, however, the way that tumescent liposuction is used by most surgeons has not been proven to give better cosmetic results.

Dr. Su's new Interactive Lipo Method takes the technique of awake liposuction and adds a few twists. By incorporating several specific techniques of patient participation during the procedure, a surgeon using the Interactive Lipo Method is able to work more effectively and can potentially create more beautiful results. Each aspect of patient participation works like a tool to give a surgeon artistic advantages in sculpting. There are many challenges in sculpting the fat layer, and each tool serves a purpose.

Dr. Su's new Interactive Lipo Method can be used on both men and women. It is versatile and can be used with great effectiveness on liposculpting all areas of the body—including the abdomen, waist, back, legs, knees, buttocks, neck, chin, and arms. The techniques incorporated in the Interactive Lipo Method can be beneficial to surgeons to greatly improve their results.

While some of the patient participation techniques in Dr. Su's method have been used by other surgeons in the past, these surgeons would be in the minority. Other parts of Dr. Su's method are quite novel. Compared to Dr. Su's method, most surgeons don't ask their patients to do much during the surgery except lie still. Some surgeons doing awake liposuction also incorporate sedatives, which make their patients unable to participate. The incorporation of all these patient participation techniques together into a cohesive method are what makes the Interactive Lipo Method novel and unique.

## ❖ Making Fat More like Wood

For a sculptor, there could not be a more difficult material to work on than the fat layer. There are many challenges and problems with sculpting the fat layer on the human body as compared to a piece of wood. These problems relate to the soft and fibrous nature of fat, which is hard to control and changes shape when a patient is lying on the table. These problems make it much more difficult for a surgeon to achieve the shape he or she desires on a patient's body, as compared to a regular sculptor. By having a patient participate with muscle tensing, the fat layer a surgeon is sculpting becomes more rigid and controllable. Liposculpting becomes easier and more predictable, like sculpting on wood.

## ❖ How Does a Patient Participate?

During the consultation, patients often nervously ask, "What will I have to do?" The answer is quite simple. A patient will be asked at different times during the surgery to get into different body positions. These positions may include lying on their back, side, face down, or sometimes leaning. They may be asked to hold themselves stable by holding the side or top of the table with their hand. At times, they will be asked to tense specific muscles. Tensing usually is held by the patient for periods lasting up to a minute. Periodically, the patient will also be asked to stand up.

Some patients have expressed concerns about whether or not they can do these things. In my experience, the vast majority can do these techniques—even patients who are older or quite out of shape are able to participate effectively. Others patients have asked whether tensing during surgery is unsafe or if it hurts. The answer is that tensing muscles makes liposuction safer, and it also helps distract patients from feeling discomfort. So let's talk about how all of this works.

### ❖ Tensing Muscles Improves Feel and Control

Unlike other sculptors, liposuction surgeons must rely on their ability to feel much more than other sculptors. While the surgeon uses one hand to move the cannula, the other hand is on the patient, feeling and controlling the fat. We'll call this the control hand. The control hand is critical in many ways. The control hand senses how deep the fat layer is. It helps the surgeon sense where the cannula is within the fat layer. It also presses the fat against the cannula to control and feed fat into the cannula.

Dr. Su's Interactive Lipo Method greatly improves the surgeon's ability to feel and control the fat layer during the sculpting process. By having a patient tense their muscles when needed, a hard surface is created below the fat layer during the surgery. This allows the surgeon to achieve a much better feel of the depth of the cannula and to hold the fat more firmly. Through better feel and control, a surgeon is able to sculpt much more accurately. Having a patient tense during the surgery is like going from sculpting on a wobbly object to sculpting on an object that is being held firmly within a clamp. No artist would try sculpting on an object that was not held firmly. Why should a liposuction surgeon?

A great example of the Interactive Lipo Method at work is when performing abdominal liposuction. The patient is lying on their back, but periodically is asked to do a "crunch". This means having a patient lie with their hands behind their head in a sit-up position but only slightly lifting the head and neck without moving the torso off the table. This stiffens the abdominal muscles sufficiently to achieve the control that is needed but does not tire a patient out. For the surgeon, it is like having a board underneath the fat instead of a waterbed. This gives the surgeon much more confidence and control in the area being sculpted.

Another major benefit of having the patient tense their muscles is the completeness that is achievable. Many surgeons are reluctant to sculpt close to the skin or muscle and end up leaving a significant amount of fat behind. If a surgeon cannot feel where fat ends and muscle begins, then there is a risk of injuring the muscle. The skin is not so easily injured. However, sculpting close to the skin requires smoothness. Having improved feel and control with a patient tensing allows a surgeon to remove the fat layer more completely near the muscle and the skin.

Having better control and feel is also very important to achieving more smoothness. As discussed earlier, the fibrous nature of fat can cause it to bunch up when the cannula is passing through it. Being able to hold the fat against a hard, tensed muscle allows it to be held firmly instead of allowing it to bunch up. This allows a surgeon to move the cannula in a smooth plane within the fat layer and remove the fat more evenly. Using an assistant to help stretch the skin in opposing directions also helps achieve the same goal. When a patient's muscles are tensed, it is also easier for the surgical assistant. In this way, the Interactive Lipo Method can truly give a surgeon the ability to achieve greater smoothness.

Tensing of the patient's muscles can be helpful for liposculpting on almost any body area. While performing liposuction on the thighs, for instance, the thighs might be held tensed together with the patient lying on their side. Another position, however, may require both thighs tensed with one leg held away from the body, resembling a Pilates pose. When doing the chin and neck, having a firm underlying surface also helps immensely and makes the procedure much safer and more accurate. As we'll see later in the discussion on sculpting of the arms, tensing of the muscles is also critical for great results in that area of the body. The Interactive Lipo Method provides the advantage that gives Dr. Su the ability to sculpt arms in a much more complete and accurate way compared to other surgeons using traditional methods. In this way, the Interactive Lipo Method allows him to create the Celebrity Arms look.

## ❖ Achieving Optimal Positioning

Having optimal positioning of the object being sculpted helps any sculptor to do better work. It is about proper ergonomics and achieving the most effective angles for sculpting efficiently. A sculptor working on wood can pick up and move an object into any angle that is needed and hold it there with clamps. A surgeon doing liposuction on an asleep or sedated patient cannot do this. Although a surgeon can employ assistants to hold a body in a certain position, it is difficult and the body would be floppy. Therefore it is not done very often. What a surgeon must do under these conditions is to sculpt from suboptimal positions or to avoid sculpting areas altogether.

A surgeon using the Interactive Lipo Method, however, can achieve the best positioning for sculpting by simply giving the patient instruction on what to do. Almost any position is possible. Some positions may require more effort for a patient to hold, so sculpting in these positions has to be done in shorter spurts.

Working on limbs can be difficult with a patient who is asleep. Because of the cylindrical shape of arms and legs, there are many more curves and angles that are needed to sculpt these areas compared to other areas of the body. Using the Interactive Lipo Method lets the surgeon place the patient in the most effective position to sculpt properly. With this ability, a surgeon can achieve results that are very smooth and complete.

For areas like the waist and back, sculpting in a three-dimensional manner around the body also requires many different angles of sculpting. Rather than having the surgeon bend and twist in difficult and fatiguing positions, a patient can be moved into multiple angles while on their side. By holding the side of the table, a patient is able to simultaneously maintain the correct position and make their body rigid.

## ❖ Standing for Visualization and Accuracy

Any artist must be able to check his or her work. In the case of liposculpting, however, this is not possible for surgeons who do not stand their patients upright. It is very difficult to accurately see or feel the thickness of the fat when a patient is lying down. In most cases, an experienced surgeon can come close. Catching small differences in areas that are uneven or not well-blended can be nearly impossible, even for the best surgeon. These are things that only appear when a patient is upright.

Areas affected by gravity, which are prone to bunching up and bulging, are even less predictable. Often the areas at the lower portion of a fat pad (closer to the ground) are the areas where bulging occurs. The degree of bulging varies unpredictably depending on the laxity of the skin. There is no way for a surgeon to tell exactly how much bulging is going to happen. Again, the only way to see what a bulge is going to do is to stand a patient upright.

For surgeons performing liposuction under general anesthesia, visualizing a patient upright is a difficult thing. A patient connected to a breathing machine cannot easily be lifted by assistants. There have been tables that tilt to almost an upright position developed to assist for this purpose, but few surgeons have them. Also, visualization would not be nearly as accurate in an upright patient when they are asleep because their muscles are relaxed.

In contrast, all doctors who perform awake liposuction without sedation can stand their patients upright. By doing this one simple thing during surgery, a surgeon can see very small inaccuracies and correct them. While giving lectures on this topic at national conferences on cosmetic surgery, I surveyed surgeons in the audience. From these surveys, I would estimate that about a third of surgeons doing awake liposuction have their patients stand to visualize results during the procedure. Why more surgeons don't adopt this method is unclear. Possibly they have not been taught that it is effective or feel that it is somehow unsafe for their patient to stand.

With the Interactive Lipo Method, the tool of having patients stand can be used throughout the entire surgery. At Artistic Lipo, we take precautions and assist the patient to ensure that standing does not present safety issues. This tool is not just about checking results at the end. I find it useful to stand patients about midway through the surgery because I can see if everything is going smoothly and as predicted. Although the shape being sculpted is visible to a large extent, it is the subtle differences that are seen. Seeing things accurately gives a surgeon the assurance to proceed more confidently.

Standing a patient more frequently has proven very beneficial in cases where the skin is looser. Looser skin can be encountered on arms, abdomens, and thigh areas. Some areas, such as the outer thigh, can be very deceptive. The area can look smooth and flat while the patient is lying down but can be uneven or have indentations when a patient stands. Catching a problem early allows a surgeon to correct it.

When a patient is standing and areas that need work are seen, a surgical pen is used to mark these areas. This is very important because the features that are seen will disappear again once the patient lies down. This process of standing, marking, and correcting is repeated until the surgery is finished.

## ❖ The Best Things in Life are Free

We live in an age where we often expect technological advances to be something fancy or scientific, like a laser used in liposuction. For patients to start getting better results in liposuction, however, an improvement in artistic skills is necessary for the surgeon performing the procedure. The Interactive Lipo Method gives surgeons quite a few tools and advantages to do their best work, and it's free. Based on the principles discussed, the Interactive Lipo Method should help any surgeon greatly improve their results, especially in the most difficult cases. The Interactive Lipo Method can be used for both men and women, and it can be applied to liposculpting of all areas of the body. With this understanding, we can now proceed to discussing the main focus of this book, which is sculpting

Celebrity Arms. Using the Interactive Lipo Method is critical in achieving this look.

# Chapter 6

Celebrity Arms: A New Ideal for Women

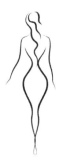

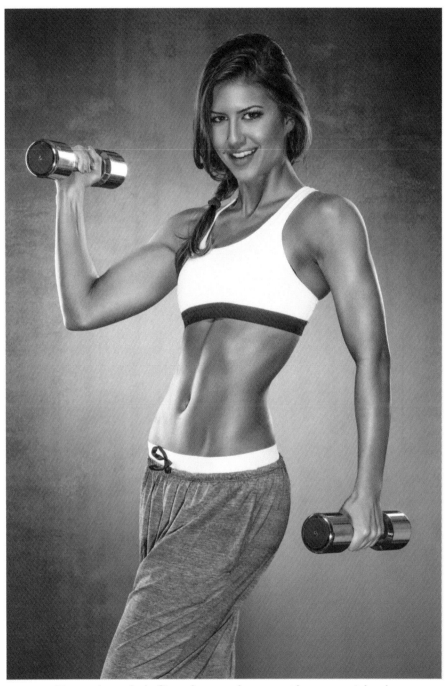

Toned and defined muscles are the new ideal.

## ❖ Having Beautiful Arms Has Become More Important

When it comes to a woman's physical beauty, there are many things that we can look at and admire. If we were to study the face alone, we could spend hours discussing the eyes, nose, and lips, just for starters. If we chose to discuss what is beautiful about a woman's body, there would also be many different aspects. Most discussions about a woman's body tend to focus on the breasts, abdomen, waist, buttocks, and legs. Traditionally, arms have not been thought of in the same way as these other body areas. This could possibly be because, in the past, the arms have not been viewed as a "sexy" part of the body.

Having great looking arms, however, is important to women for a number of reasons. The arms, even if they are not the main focus of beauty for a woman, do enhance her beauty in other ways. Slimmer arms can make a woman look slimmer overall. Having toned and defined arms gives a woman an overall fit look. Having great-looking arms also enhances the look of the breasts and upper back. Most women have at least some concern about their arms and how to make them look better—just ask any woman who has thought about wearing a sleeveless dress.

In the past three decades, there has been a consistent movement towards fitness for both sexes. Women in the '80s and '90s were focused on general fitness through aerobic routines. Through aerobics, women were actively trying to get slimmer and more toned in their abs and legs. Since the '90s, in addition to developing the lower body, there has been a shift to strength training and developing arms, shoulders, and backs. There are a lot more women today who are actively lifting weights to develop their muscle tone than in the past. More women today are into fitness and bodybuilding competitions than in previous decades. A toned and athletic figure is now much more desirable than it has ever been in the past.

## ❖ Celebrity Arms—A Glimpse of the New Ideal

When it comes to beauty, our ideals often come from what the tabloid magazines and beauty magazines show us. Celebrities from movies and television programs often influence fashion, hair styles, and even the body types that are considered the most desirable. Whether a celebrity is actually creating a new trend or following a current trend is unimportant. What is clear is that when the media begins to focus on celebrities for certain aspects of their beauty, a new ideal can be defined.

One of the trends of the last decade is that women started getting noticed for their arms by the media. Some of the earlier celebrities to be singled out were Kelly Ripa, Jennifer Aniston, and Angelina Jolie. After Kelly Ripa became so well-known for her beautiful arms, it was not unusual to hear other women state that they wanted "Kelly Ripa Arms". Another surprising trend was seen when Michelle Obama became the First Lady. It seemed that the media was obsessed with her beautiful arms and was more interested in talking about her arms than her agenda. The internet also was flooded with workout and training videos about "How to Get Michelle Obama Arms." The trend continues, and some of the celebrities that are currently admired for their arms are Jessica Biel and Jennifer Garner. If you do an internet search for "beautiful arms," pictures of these celebrities and others will appear.

## ❖ Celebrity Arms Defined

So, what is it about the arms of the celebrities we have mentioned that has the media and the general public so enthralled? There are several commonalities, and it is in those commonalities that we can define what the Celebrity Arms ideal is. Celebrity Arms are beautiful because they are slim, shapely, and toned. Having only slim arms does not make these arms beautiful. It is the combination of slimness along with the curves and contours of well-toned muscles that creates the Celebrity Arms look.

Perhaps the most important feature that stands out in the Celebrity Arms look is a well-toned and defined shoulder. A toned shoulder has an outward rounded shape which cuts inward about midway down the upper arm. The shoulder muscle is separated by a groove or indentation where it meets the biceps muscle. There is also another groove that borders the lower edge of the shoulder muscle where it meets the triceps muscle. Having the individual shapes and contours of all three muscles in the upper arm is what gives the arm its beautiful shape. A slim arm with both defined arm and shoulder muscles creates the Celebrity Arms look.

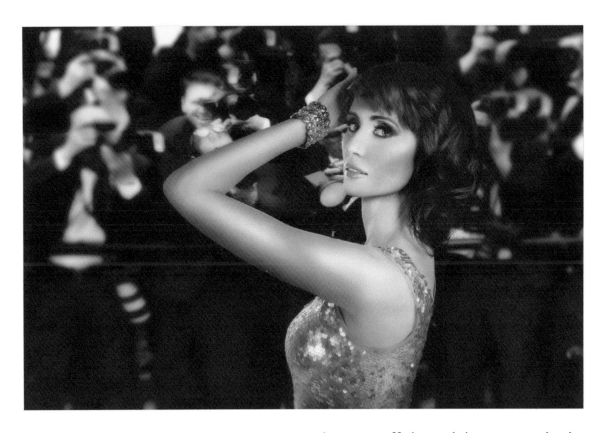

Professional spokesmodel Oksana Boss showing off the Celebrity Arms look.

## ❖ Other Ideals of Arm Beauty

Although many women today would love to have the defined and toned Celebrity Arms look, this is, of course, not for everyone. In the United States, the Celebrity Arms look is quite popular. In most of South America, however, women are still admired for having a fuller and rounder appearance in most body areas. Latina women are known for their full bottoms and breasts, and the arms naturally follow this trend as well. In Europe and the United States, the fashion industry also has a different ideal. Female models are known for being tall and thin. Having straight, thin arms with no muscle definition is the desired ideal in the fashion industry.

# Chapter 7

## The Challenge of Achieving Celebrity Arms

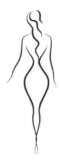

## ❖ Hard Work and Exercise Do Not Guarantee Celebrity Arms

Women today really want the slimmed, toned, and defined look of Celebrity Arms. Therefore, it not surprising that women are exercising their arms much more than in the past. Unfortunately, doing more arm and shoulder exercises does not guarantee that women will get the results they are looking for. On the contrary, most women who have tried to achieve the Celebrity Arms look through exercise have failed.

If we look at what women are doing to achieve this look, we see that there are more things being done than ever before. It's no longer just aerobic routines or lifting weights. Women these days are doing many different types of fitness routines including boot camps, boxing, and mud run races. There are many different arm routines that vary from lifting low weight with high repetitions to doing fewer repetitions with heavy weight. There are also routines using elastic bands, kettlebells, and even heavy ropes. Every trainer promises to have the secret arm routine to get ideal, defined arms. Even some of the best female trainers (who are in terrific shape) don't have slim and defined arms.

What women are achieving through all these types of exercise is arm strengthening, but not necessarily better muscle definition. Every woman who works out her arms regularly will strengthen her arms. She will develop larger and stronger muscles. Most women who want to have the Celebrity Arms look already have enough muscle because of their exercise routines. So, why aren't all these women achieving their goal of seeing muscle definition?

## ❖ The Problem Is Not Muscle, It Is Fat

The definition of the shoulder, biceps, and triceps muscles is created by subtle muscle shapes and the grooves in between these muscles. In order to see these muscle features, there cannot be much fat overlying the muscle. Everywhere on the body, there is a layer of fat between the skin and muscle. On the female arm, it is this layer of fat that hides much of the muscle definition. Because the contours of the arm muscles in women are not large, it takes only a quarter-inch thickness of fat to obscure the muscle contours in many women.

There is a big difference between men and women when it comes to arm definition. Men have a much lower percentage of body fat compared to women, and this is more apparent in the arms. Most women have a layer of fat on their arms that can be a quarter-inch to a half-inch thick, compared to men who often have almost no fat in this area. That is why men can achieve definition fairly easily in their arms when they work out, but women have a difficult time.

So why doesn't exercising the arms burn away this fat layer on the arms? Contrary to what many people think, working out specific body areas does not get rid of fat in that area. It is not possible to target specific areas of fat to get rid of. Fat is not burned just in the area of the muscle being exercised. Fat is burned from throughout the entire body during exercise. That is why women don't see defined arms just by working out. Working out the arms builds muscle, but does little to reduce the fat layer.

Many women who work out their arms rigorously report looking worse. This is possible because when the arm muscles strengthen, they enlarge. If the fat layer stays the same, then a larger muscle underneath can lead to a bulkier look.

## ❖ Diets Are Not Very Useful Either

Diets have also not been very effective in helping women achieve the Celebrity Arms look. Dieting is a good means of losing weight and getting rid of fat in general. The fat that is lost cannot be targeted at a specific area on the body. A woman will be slimmer overall. However, she may not see any improvement on her arms. Everyone is designed a bit differently from a genetic standpoint, and some women tend to keep their arm fat more stubbornly than others.

Many women who want the slim and defined look on their arms are already close to their ideal body weight. Losing more weight to try to get rid of that small amount of fat on the arms often has unwanted effects. Instead of fat leaving the arms, a woman may see fat lost in areas like the breasts, buttocks, and face, which would have an overall negative effect on her appearance.

## ❖ Traditional Cosmetic Surgery Is Not a Solution

In their pursuit of achieving more beautiful arms, women in the last decade have been resorting to cosmetic surgery more than ever before. Whether it is because of the trend seen with celebrity's arms is unclear, but it has been well documented. In their annual report "2013 Plastic Surgery Statistics Report", the American Society for Plastic Surgery (ASPS) revealed a startling fact. In the past 13 years, they reported an overall increase in cosmetic arm surgeries of more than 4000 percent—that is, over forty times what was seen in the previous decade.[1]

When it comes to cosmetic or plastic surgery, however, the existing traditional surgeries only target the lower "underhang" portion of the arm. These surgeries have only helped to slim arms. Nothing that has existed until now has been able to give a woman the Celebrity Arms look. No surgery in the past has been able to achieve both slimness and muscle definition in the arm and shoulder region.

The two surgeries that are being referred to as traditional cosmetic surgeries of the arm are brachioplasty and liposuction. Although the goal of both of these surgeries is to improve the appearance of the underhang of the arm, the two types of surgery are vastly different. Each surgery approaches the problem area in a very different way. Depending on the patient, one surgery may be more appropriate than the other. In some cases, both types of surgery may be used in conjunction.

---

[1] American Society for Plastic Surgery, "2013 Plastic Surgery Statistics Report", (http://www.plasticsurgery.org/Documents/news-resources/statistics/2013-statistics/plastic-surgery-statistics-full-report-2013.pdf), 7.

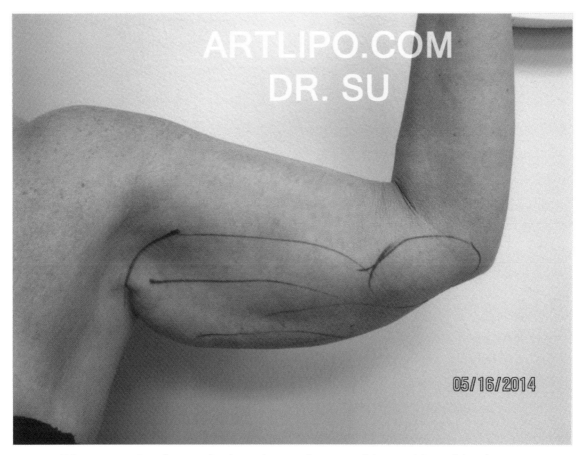

Photograph of a typical patient who would need brachioplasty
because her arm has too much sagging skin and fat to be
a good candidate for the Celebrity Arms look.

## ❖ Brachioplasty Is for Loose Skin

Brachioplasty (which is commonly known as an *arm lift* or *arm tuck*) is the best type of surgery for a woman who has a large area of sagging skin and fat on the lower portion of the arm (see photograph on preceding page). A brachioplasty surgically removes this sag by cutting both the skin and the fat away. The area is then stitched back together, leaving a linear scar on the arm. This can be compared to the more common *tummy tuck* (called an abdominoplasty) which is done in a very similar fashion and leaves a linear scar along the line of the sag of the fat pad at the bottom of the abdomen. The goal of a brachioplasty is to get rid of the lower arm hang. This procedure does not affect the upper or side portions of the arm in any way that would reveal muscle definition. Therefore, it cannot achieve toned arms or shoulders and cannot provide the Celebrity Arms look.

## ❖ Traditional Liposuction Treats the Underhang of the Arm

Traditional arm liposuction has also been a very popular surgery. The area being treated is typically the underhang of the arm only. Ninety-five percent of surgeons never treat beyond this area. Patients who would benefit from this type of surgery usually have a thick area of fat hanging on the underside of the arm. Surgeons performing arm liposuction sometimes blend the sculpting into the side of the arm. However, full liposuction of the sides, front, and top of the arms and shoulders has been discouraged by many liposuction experts and teachers for different reasons. Surgeons are

**BEFORE**

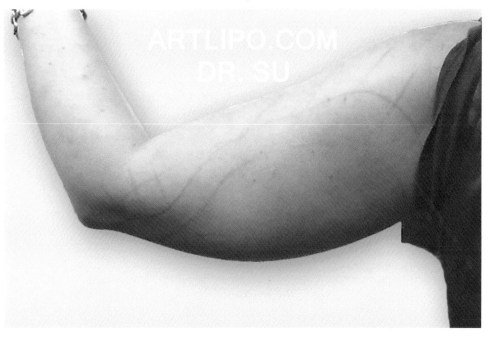

**AFTER**

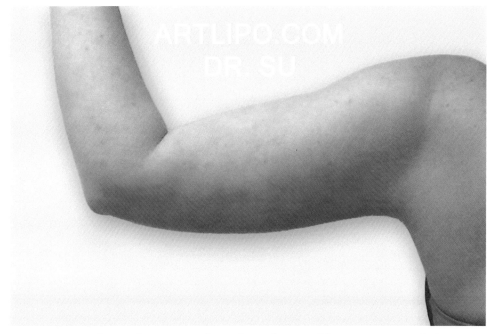

Before and after photographs of traditional liposuction of the arms with some blending into the sides and shoulders. Although slimmer, this arm does not have the definition of the Celebrity Arms look.

taught throughout their training to avoid these areas. The difficulty level and potential for irregularities is the main reason surgeons are dissuaded from sculpting the sides of the arms and shoulders. Therefore, traditional liposuction has never been a method of achieving the Celebrity Arms look.

# Chapter 8

## Creating Celebrity Arms Using Dr. Su's New Interactive Lipo Method

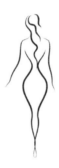

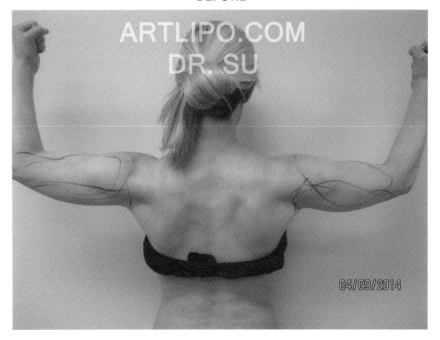

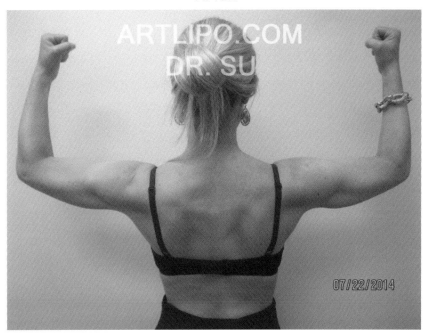

Before and after photographs of a patient who had the Celebrity Arms look created by Dr. Su, using his Interactive Lipo Method.

## ❖ What is Unique about Celebrity Arms Liposculpting?

Celebrity Arms liposculpting is a brand-new concept that very few people know about, including cosmetic surgeons. It is about taking liposuction of the arms to a completely different level. Surgeons are no longer restricted to only the underhang of the arm, like traditional liposuction. Celebrity Arms sculpting involves the entire arm and shoulder on all surfaces in a 360-degree manner. The sculpting is blended to the edges of the upper back, as well as to the beginning of the forearm. This is a full circumferential sculpting of the arms. The photographs on the previous page and the next page illustrate the extent of the sculpted areas, as shown by the pre-surgical markings in the before photos.

Celebrity Arms liposculpting goes way beyond just sculpting in a circumferential manner. The difference with Celebrity Arms sculpting is the degree to which the fat is sculpted and the intricate contours revealed. Celebrity Arms sculpting is not just about removing some fat. It is about removing fat very completely and skillfully and following the curves and shapes of the muscles. This results in the appearance that the patient has been working out for months. It is about taking an arm that is lacking in definition or outwardly bulging, and sculpting away the fat to reveal the natural contours of the muscles and create a much slimmer profile. Comparing Celebrity Arms liposculpting to traditional liposuction of the arm would be like comparing a three-dimensional sculpture to a flat two-dimensional drawing.

**BEFORE**

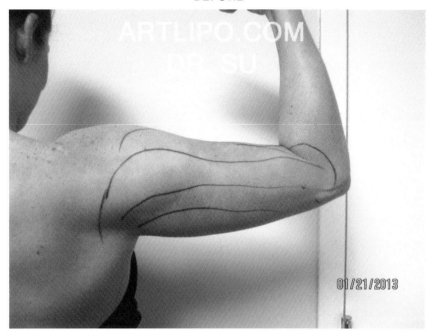

**AFTER**

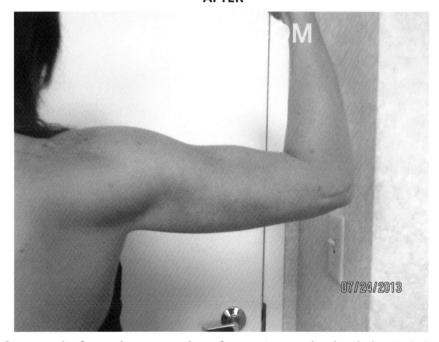

Before and after photographs of a patient who had the Celebrity Arms look created by Dr. Su, using his Interactive Lipo Method.

## ❖ Why Hasn't This Been Done Before?

Liposuction has been around for over thirty years, and in that time, many things have been tried. Because of the difficulty involved in surgery, some things have succeeded, while others have failed. Sometimes, a small adjustment such as a new instrument may be needed before new things become possible. Other times, however, a radical change in approach is needed. To create Celebrity Arms, a whole different approach was needed.

Creating the Celebrity Arms look has definitely been tried in the past by countless surgeons before me. It is only natural for an artistic surgeon to want to achieve a fully sculpted arm and not just a thinning of the underhang. It is clear, however, that very few surgeons are currently attempting anything close to full circumferential sculpting of the arms. By conservative estimates, probably less than five percent of all surgeons doing liposuction have attempted this. These estimates are based on polls I conducted of surgeons attending lectures I have given on this topic at both the ASCOP and AACS (two of the largest cosmetic surgery organizations in the United States). Also, if you do an extensive search on the internet for keywords such as "full arm liposuction," "circumferential arm liposuction," or "high definition arm liposuction," you will find very few examples of before and after pictures actually showing fully sculpted arms. Of the examples that I have seen, the sculpting is not as smooth or complete as could be desired.

The reason that cosmetic surgeons are not performing full arm sculpting or Celebrity Arms sculpting is because it is not being taught. On the contrary, surgeons are being taught in their training and at conferences that circumferential arm sculpting should not be done. Much of the experience that has led to this line of thought has been carried forth from prior decades. From the 1980s until 2000, most liposuction surgeries were being performed under general anesthesia. Limitations of liposuction being done on a patient who is asleep are much greater than in an awake, participating patient, as we have discussed in earlier chapters. These limitations also apply to surgeries where the patient is awake but not asked to participate.

Because of these limitations, there has been significantly more difficulty in producing a beautiful result when it comes to full sculpting of the arms and shoulders. Lack of consistency and a high chance of unwanted irregularities are what led the cosmetic surgery community to warn against sculpting the arm beyond the underhang. Although there are always difficulties in doing liposuction of any part of the body, these difficulties are greatly magnified when it comes to doing full liposuction of the arms.

Going back to the earlier discussion about the difficulties of liposuction—all of them come into play here. The sides of the arms and shoulders are thinner areas compared to other areas of the body that are sculpted. Working in a thinner area means that even small irregularities in sculpting will easily be seen. These irregularities cannot be masked. Also, these areas are more fibrous in nature than most areas of the body, which makes it difficult to move a cannula smoothly. Without smooth movement of a cannula, a smooth final result is not possible. Another problem is the cylindrical shape of the arm, which needs to be sculpted in a 360 degree fashion. Going around such a sharply curved surface introduces significant difficulty. Finally, the shape of the arm is not just a smooth cylinder.

Instead, it is a cylinder with additional specific curves and grooves of the different muscle groups. Trying to follow those curves and grooves in sculpting is next to impossible unless they can be felt while the muscles are tensed.

## ❖ The Interactive Lipo Method Makes Celebrity Arms Possible

If there was a part of the body in which the benefits of the Interactive Lipo Method was exemplified, it would be in creating Celebrity Arms. During the development of the Interactive Lipo Method, it became clear to me how different my method of performing arm surgery was when compared to other surgeons. Other surgeons have their patients on their backs, often working from one or two fixed positions. Their patients are either asleep or awake, but in either case their arms are relaxed. In contrast, I have my patients in many different positions. My patients are on their backs for some positions, but they are also on their sides and sometimes in a leaning position. With each body position, the arms also have multiple positions. The arms may be bent at different angles or held straight. In addition, the arms are often held firm or tensed, with the hand gripping the sides of the table or gripping the other hand. The effect is a very stable and versatile surface of the arm to work on.

The benefit of having so many positions with the patient actively tensing their arm and shoulder muscles is to gain the advantages that any good sculptor needs to succeed. Those advantages, which have been discussed earlier, are "feel and control," "optimal positioning," and "visualization."

Having the firmness of tensed muscles underneath the fat gives a surgeon a huge advantage by feeling the fat layer accurately. Grasping that fat layer on the arm to stabilize it is also significantly easier with the muscles tensed. By stabilizing and feeling the fat more accurately, the cannula can be passed back and forth more smoothly. This helps to overcome the significant difficulties of the arm being more fibrous. The improved feel also gives a great advantage in working smoothly within the thin layer of fat on the arm. Irregularities, therefore, are significantly less likely. Also, the tensing of the muscles allows a surgeon to feel the contour and grooves of the muscles in the arm and shoulder. Without this component, a surgeon would have a difficult time revealing these features accurately.

Achieving optimal positioning also allows a surgeon to work in the most effective way, just like a sculptor who needs to work from many different angles. It is more effective to move the sculpture into the correct position instead of trying to sculpt from an angle that is difficult for the artist. Likewise, the surgeon needs many directions and angles to work from to cover all the different angles and surfaces of the arm.

Seeing the contours and shapes being created on the arm is very difficult for a surgeon when a patient is lying on their back. This is not a flat surface that has to be visualized, but a full 360 degree cylindrical shape. In the lying position, gravity distorts the shape of the arm significantly and makes it difficult to determine if the sculpting is accurate. It is very helpful, therefore, to have a patient sit up periodically and have her flex her muscles from all different positions. This gives a surgeon the ability to accurately see the shape that is being revealed on the arm muscles. It then gives the surgeon the ability to know exactly where more sculpting needs to be done. This takes the liposculpting from being a guessing game, as it is in traditional liposuction, to being more objective and precise.

If it were not for the Interactive Lipo Method, Celebrity Arms liposculpting would not be possible. The results would not be consistent. The difficulties would be too great to achieve smooth and beautiful results. It is appropriate, therefore, that surgeons who are not using Interactive Lipo avoid sculpting the arm fully. For those surgeons with more experience and skill, however, using the Interactive Lipo Method will allow something that was not previously possible. Finally, there is a method that will allow women to get the shape and contours that they have always wanted in their arms!

## ❖ How Is Celebrity Arms Sculpting Done?

As discussed throughout this book, Interactive Lipo is performed with a patient fully awake and alert. Only local anesthetic infused into the area being sculpted is used. The only instrumentation that is used is the same type of suction cannula that all surgeons must use to remove fat no matter what type of liposuction they are doing. No additional lasers, ultrasound, or power-assisted devices are needed or used. Strong sculpting skills are the main tools needed to achieve great results.

To achieve the Celebrity Arms look, it also takes a dedicated patient who is prepared to participate, as this makes a huge difference in the results that are created. In my experience, all the patients that I have performed

Celebrity Arms liposculpting on could easily do what was required. I've had patients compare the tensing and holding of positions to Pilates. The Celebrity Arms surgery only takes about an hour per side, and time passes by rather quickly. Often my patients are engaged in conversation with myself or my nurse throughout the surgery.

From a tolerability standpoint, Celebrity Arms liposculpting is generally better tolerated than most other areas of the body. It is not always comfortable, and there are some short-lived painful pinches, which most patients will feel at times. Though most patients are somewhat nervous initially, most tell me that it was not too bad or that it was not anything like what they were expecting. The recovery is quick, but still involves a few days of soreness and taking it easy. Patients wear a sleeve-like compression garment for two weeks. The results are immediate, but some swelling will take up to a few months to resolve.

## ❖ Who Is a Good Candidate?

Most women who do not have overtly loose or sagging skin on their arms can be a good candidate for Celebrity Arms liposculpting. Those with looser skin may need a brachioplasty. Obviously, patients with smooth, firm, elastic skin will be the ones with the tightest skin afterwards. I usually advise patients to come into my office for a consultation or to send photos via email or text if they live far away. This ensures that we can give the best advice.

As far as thickness of fat, I can treat a wide range of patients. The patients with thicker fat on their arms will have the most dramatic results. Very thin patients who don't have a lot of fat, however, can still often see a nice difference in muscle definition. Those patients with good muscle tone and skin tone with a moderate to large amount of fat are the ideal body type to get the best results in both shape and skin quality. The next chapter shows examples of all these different body types.

## ❖ How Do I Get Celebrity Arms?

The best way to get started is to contact our office, Artistic Lipo, by phone or email. We will set up a consultation at our office or over the phone. Since we have patients flying in from different states and countries, we are used to setting up the accommodations for our visiting patients. If you can't come into the office for a consultation, we will need you to send photos for Dr. Su to evaluate. Our staff will be able to assist you when you call. We look forward to hearing from you!

# Chapter 9

## Celebrity Arms Gallery

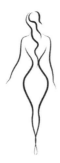

# Group A

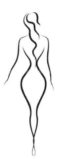

## Patients with Light to Medium Fat Layer and No Skin Sagging

**BEFORE**

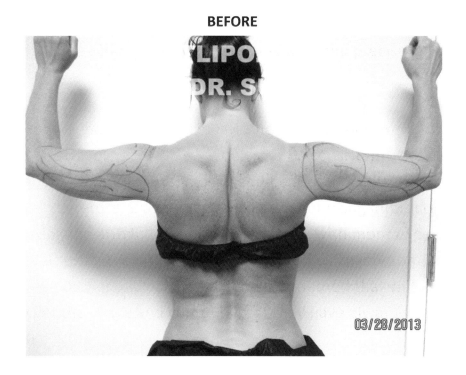

**AFTER**

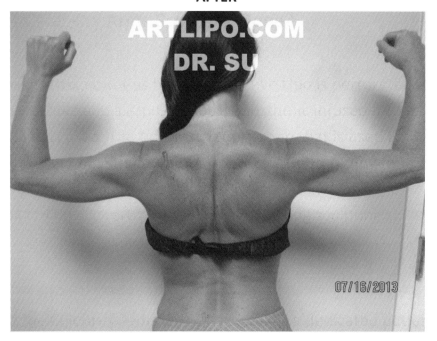

**Case 1** - A patient in her thirties who is very active and fit but who had just a small to medium layer of fat. She looks slimmer and has significant definition and curves afterwards.

**BEFORE**

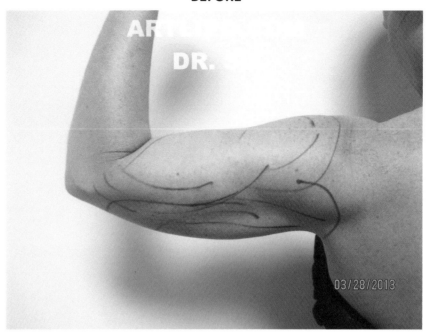

**AFTER**

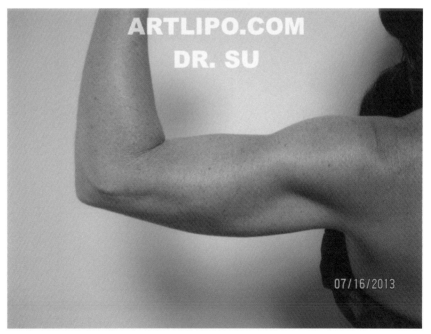

**Case 1** - continued

**BEFORE**

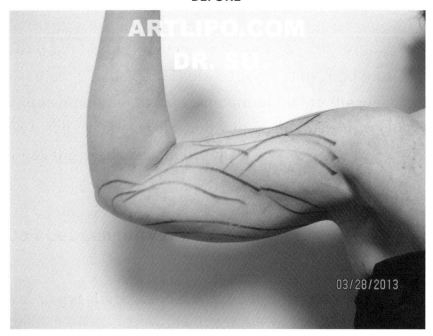

**AFTER**

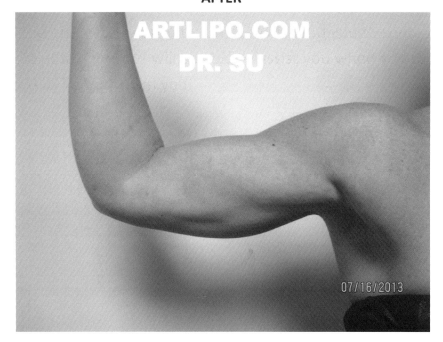

**Case 1** - continued

**BEFORE**

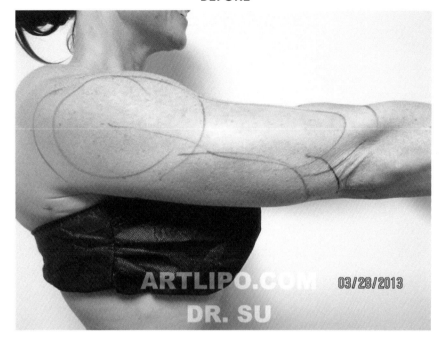

**AFTER**

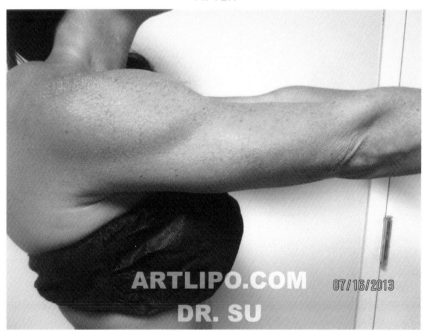

**Case 1** - continued

**BEFORE**

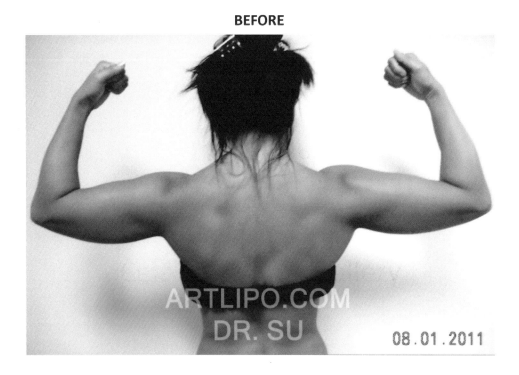

**AFTER**

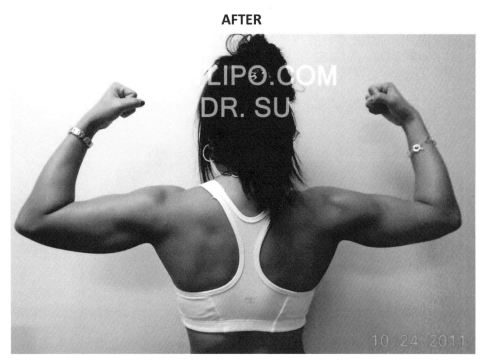

**Case 2** – A patient in her twenties who works out at the gym but was unable to get rid of the fat. Because of this, she could not achieve the definition she desired. Her result is a much more lean and defined look.

**BEFORE**

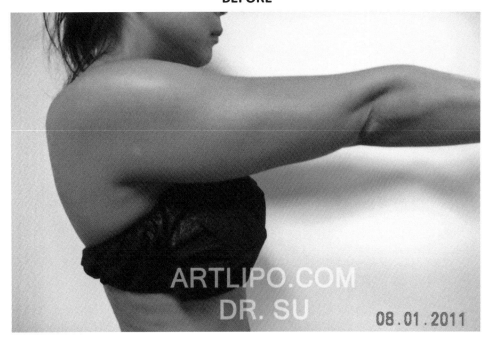

**AFTER**

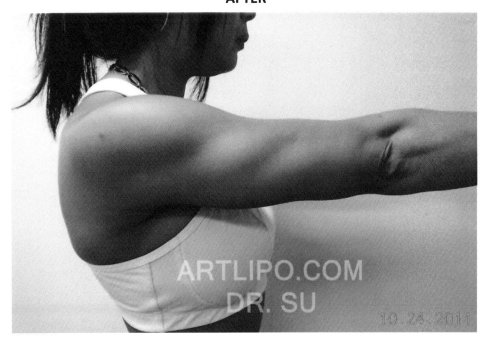

**Case 2** – continued

**BEFORE**

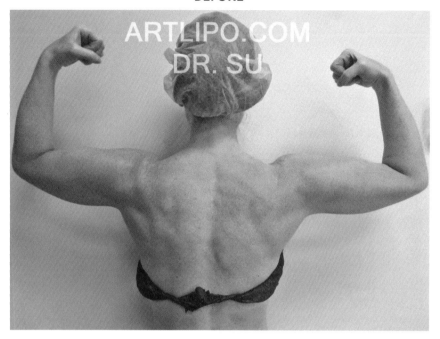

**AFTER**

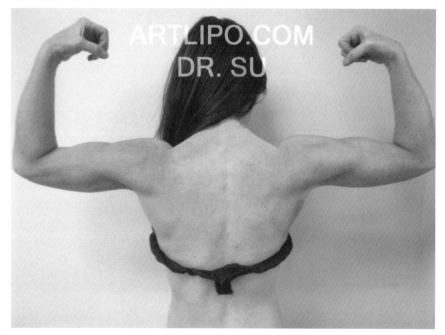

**Case 3** – A patient in her thirties with fair definition, but who had a medium layer of fat. She has slimming and stunning definition after Celebrity Arms sculpting.

**BEFORE**

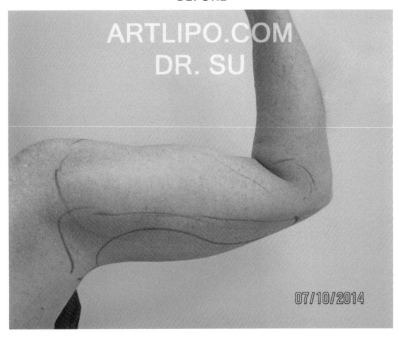

**AFTER**

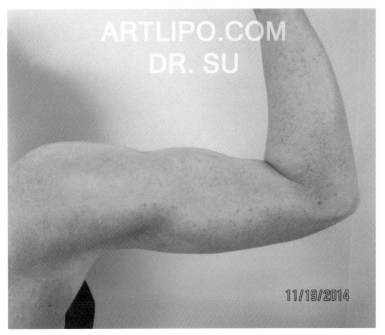

**Case 3** - continued

**BEFORE**

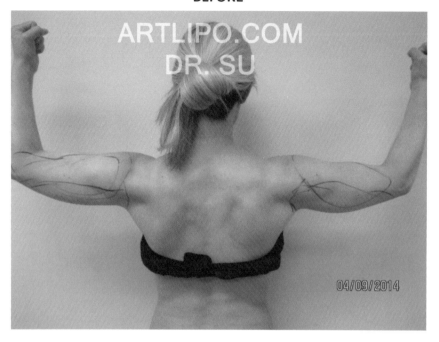

**AFTER**

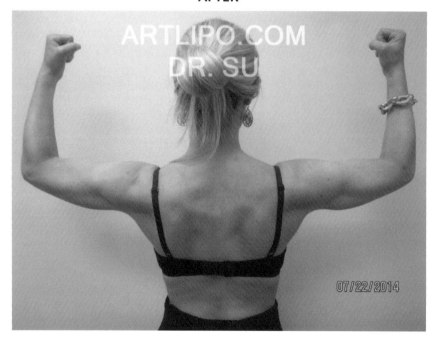

**Case 4** – A patient in her early thirties who works out regularly but wanted slimmer arms and more definition, which she has after Celebrity Arms sculpting.

**BEFORE**

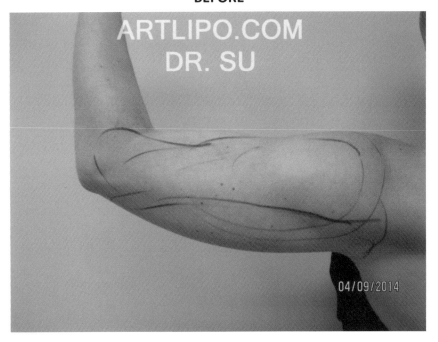

**AFTER**

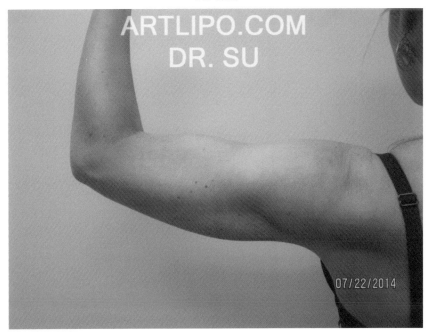

**Case 4** - continued

**BEFORE**

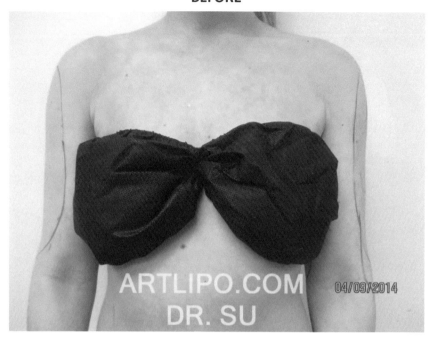

**AFTER**

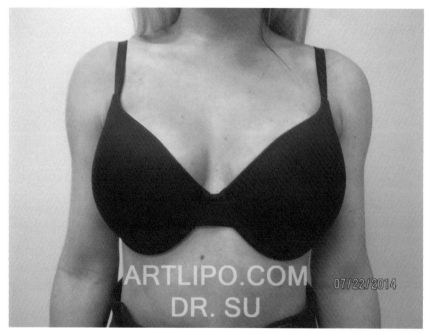

**Case 4** – continued. In this view of the patient, the dramatic difference in the frontal contours of her entire figure can easily be seen.

**BEFORE**

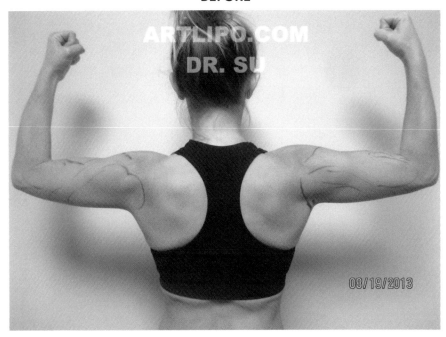

**AFTER**

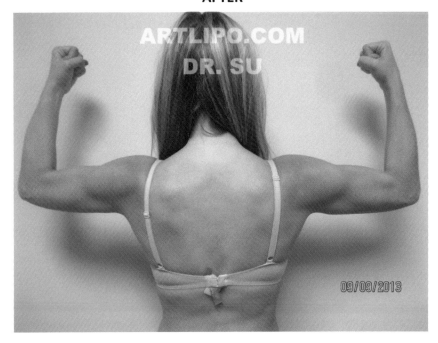

**Case 5** – This patient in her late twenties was already slim and toned, but wished to have more definition than she could get by just working out.

**BEFORE**

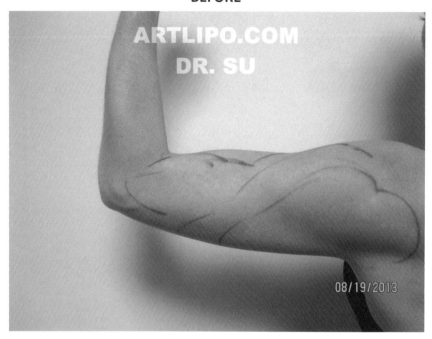

**AFTER**

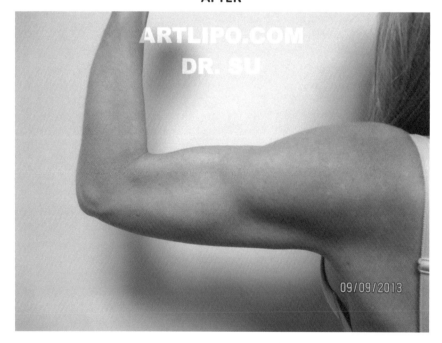

**Case 5** - continued

**BEFORE**

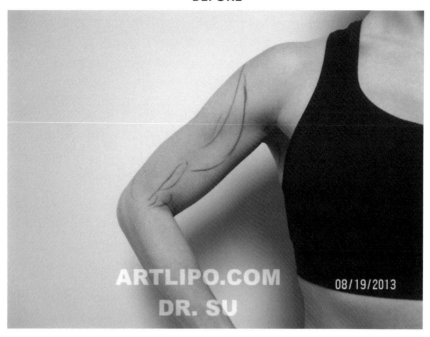

**AFTER**

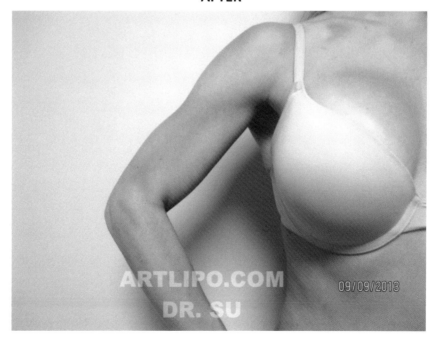

**Case 5** – continued. In this view of the patient, it can be seen how the shoulder definition is also improved in an active state.

**BEFORE**

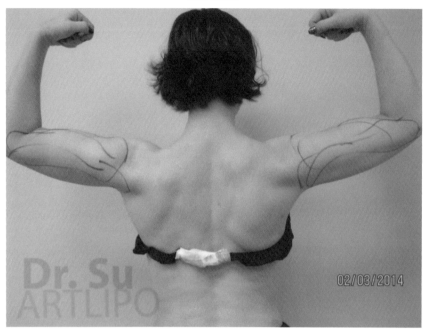

**AFTER**

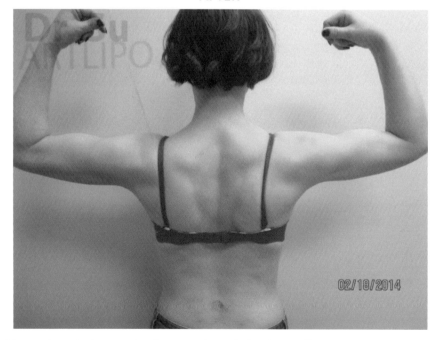

**Case 6** – This patient in her early thirties already had excellent tone in her muscles, but she had a small layer of fat. Her results give her a slimmer and more toned appearance.

**BEFORE**

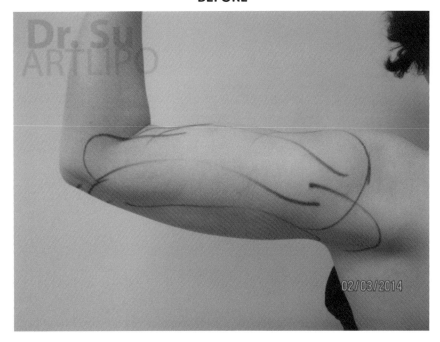

**AFTER**

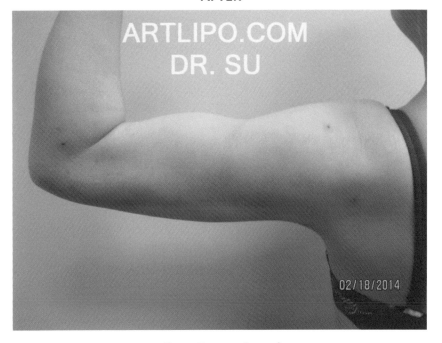

**Case 6** - continued

**BEFORE**

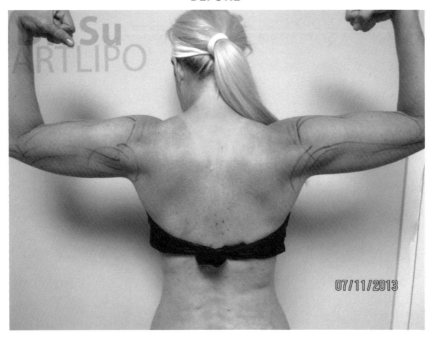

**AFTER**

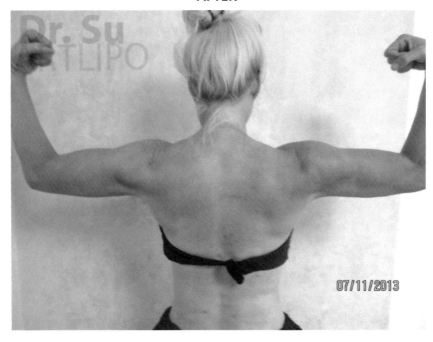

**Case 7** – A patient in her twenties with a moderate layer of fat. The after photo was taken immediately after surgery. The incisions have been blurred in the after photograph, but the results were immediate.

**BEFORE**

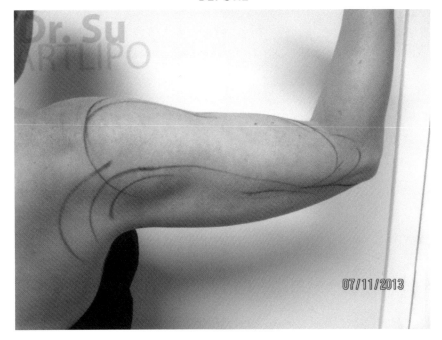

**AFTER**

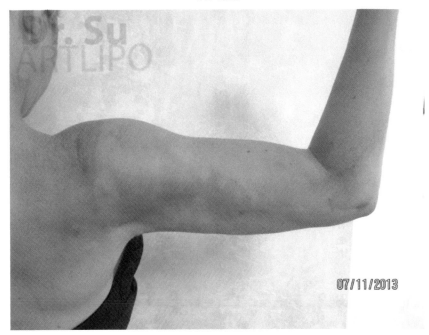

**Case 7** – continued

**BEFORE**

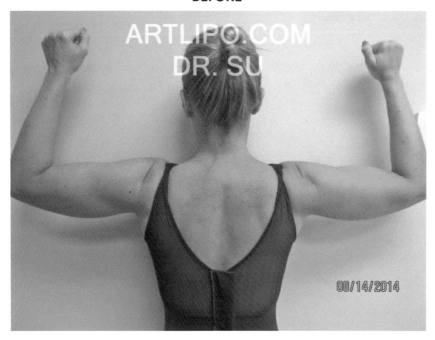

**AFTER**

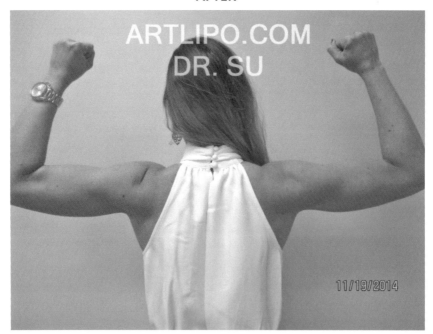

**Case 8** – This patient in her late twenties had very developed muscles with a small layer of fat. After Interactive Lipo, her arms now have a slimmer and toned appearance.

**BEFORE**

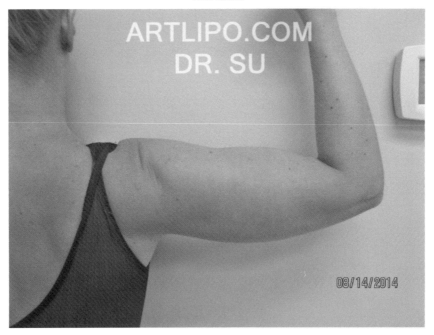

**AFTER**

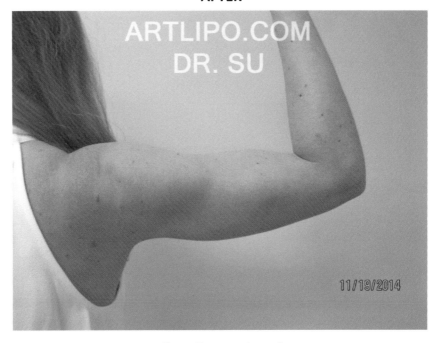

**Case 8** – continued

**BEFORE**

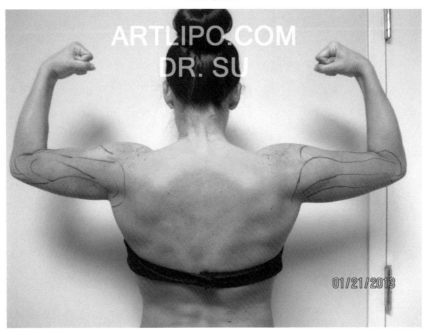

**AFTER**

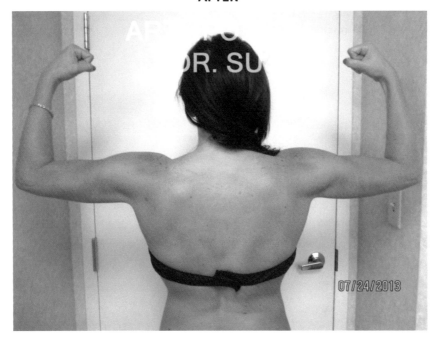

**Case 9** – This patient in her thirties was fit, but she had a medium layer of fat hiding her arm definition. Her result is slimmer and more toned arms.

**BEFORE**

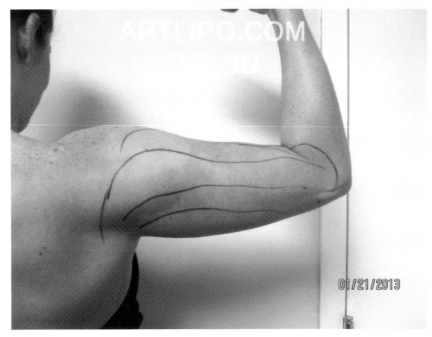

**AFTER**

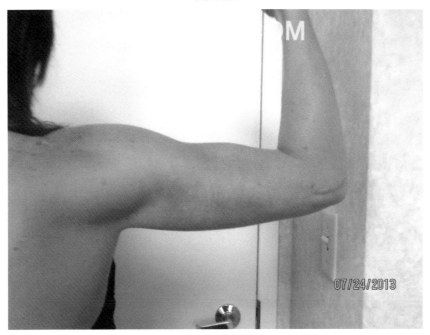

**Case 9** – continued

**BEFORE**

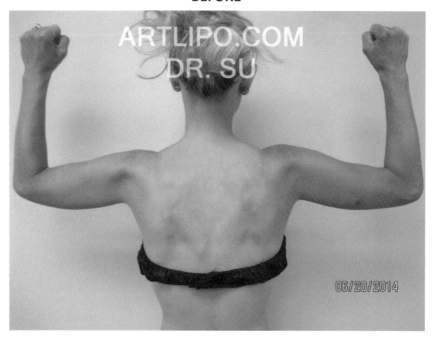

**AFTER**

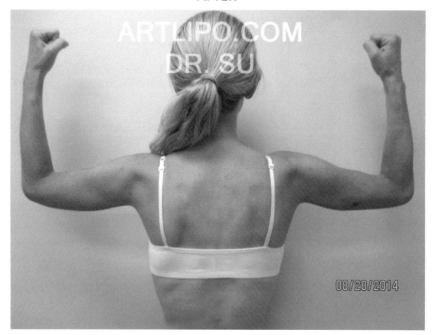

**Case 10** – A patient in her thirties with a very slim shape, but little visible muscle tone. After sculpting a medium layer of fat, her toned muscles are revealed.

**BEFORE**

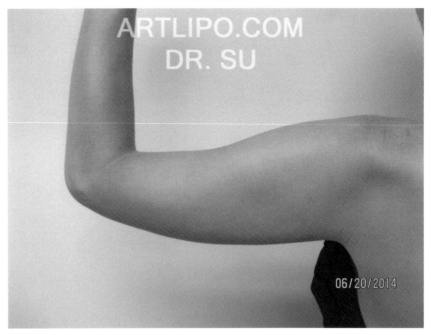

**AFTER**

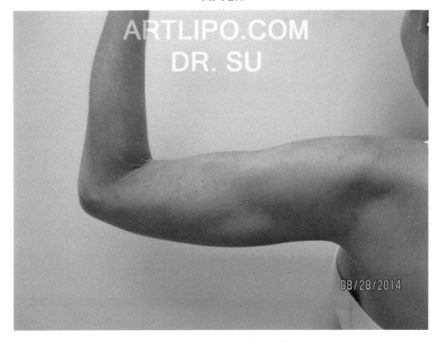

**Case 10** – continued

**BEFORE**

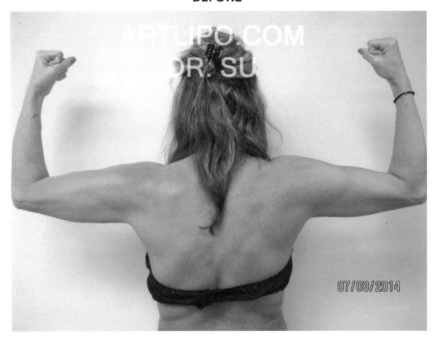

**AFTER**

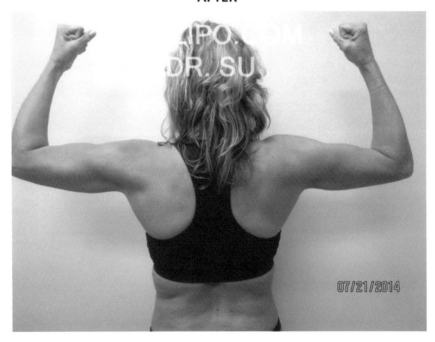

**Case 11** – A patient in her forties with vague muscle shape and definition. After sculpting away a medium layer of fat, she has a very nice shape and a toned appearance.

**BEFORE**

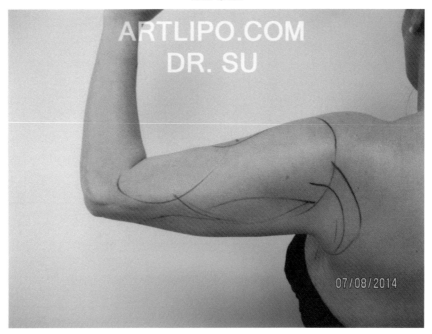

**AFTER**

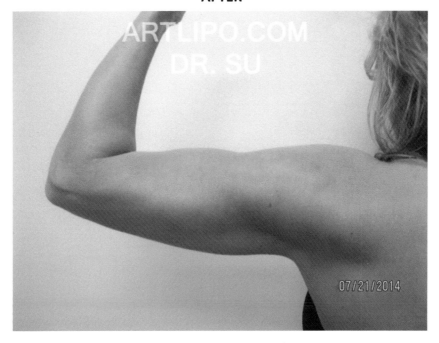

**Case 11** – continued

# Group B

Patients with Large Fat Layer and No Skin Sagging

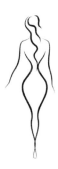

**BEFORE**

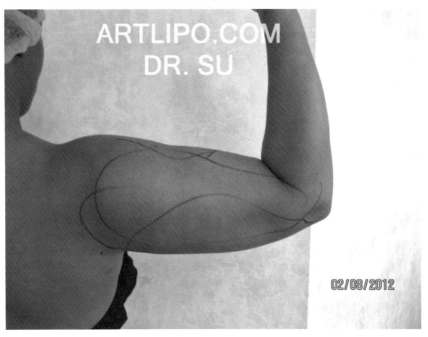

**AFTER**

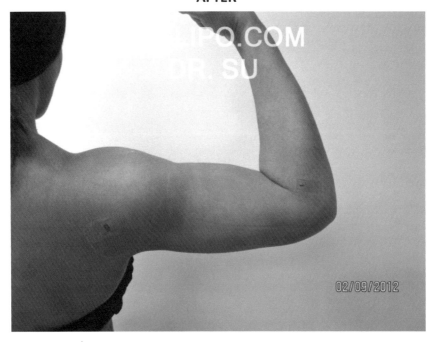

**Case 12** – This patient in her forties had very thick fat layer with a fairly even distribution. After her sculpting, she is much thinner and has great shape and curves in her arms.

**BEFORE**

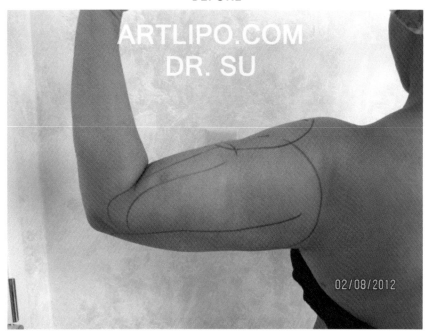

**AFTER**

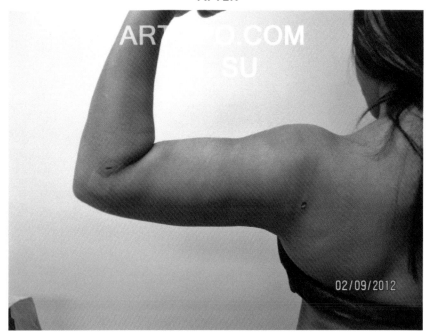

**Case 12** – continued

**BEFORE**

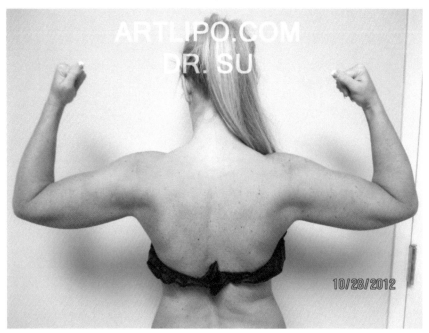

**AFTER**

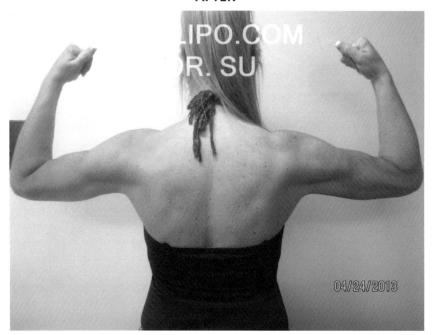

**Case 13** – This patient in her forties had a very thick layer of fat in an even distribution. After sculpting, she looks very thin, toned, and shapely.

**BEFORE**

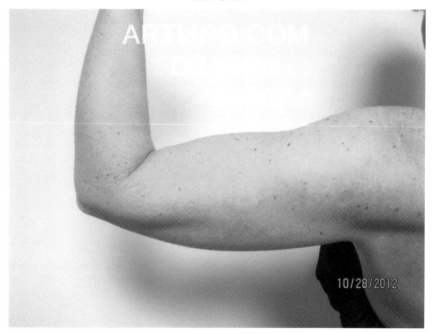

**AFTER**

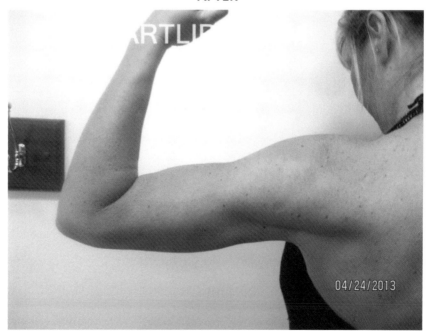

**Case 13** – continued

**BEFORE**

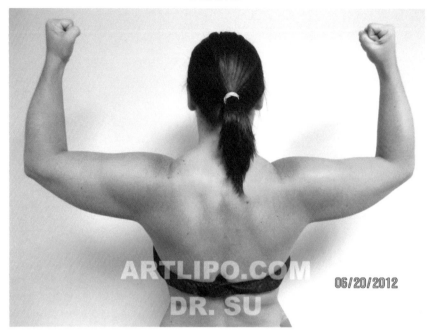

**AFTER**

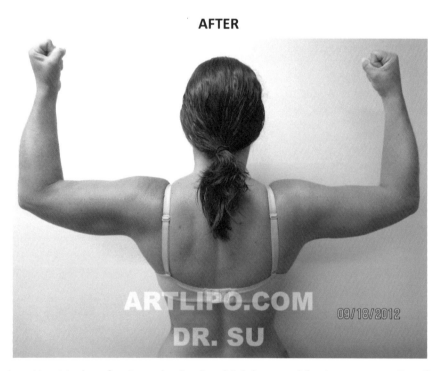

**Case 14** – A patient in her forties who had a thick layer of fat in an even distribution. After sculpting, her arms appear slimmer and more of her muscle shape is revealed.

**BEFORE**

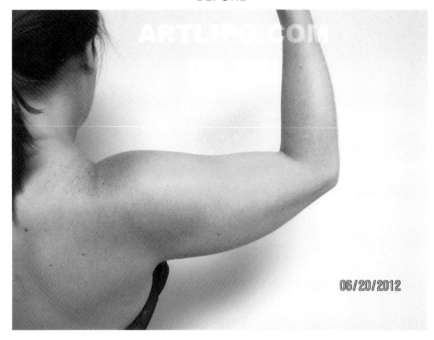

**AFTER**

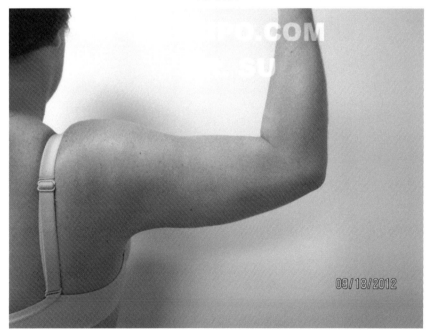

**Case 14** – continued

**BEFORE**

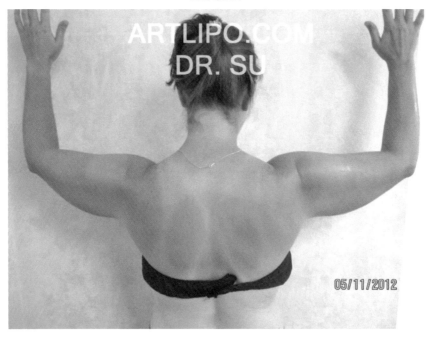

**AFTER**

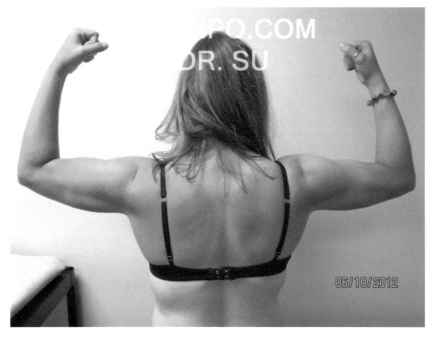

**Case 15** - A patient in her forties with thick fat, distributed heavier in the arm underhang. After sculpting, she shows very good muscle definition and is much slimmer.

**BEFORE**

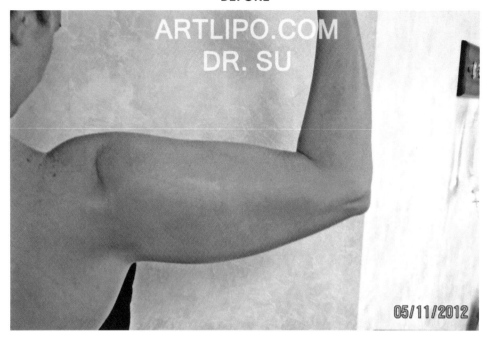

**AFTER**

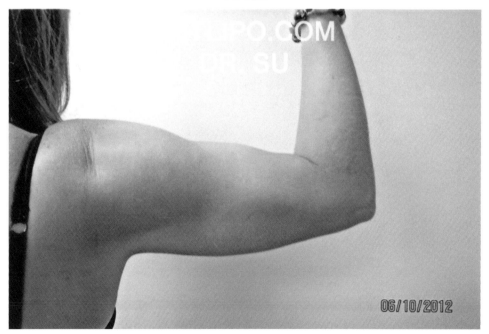

**Case 15** – continued

**BEFORE**

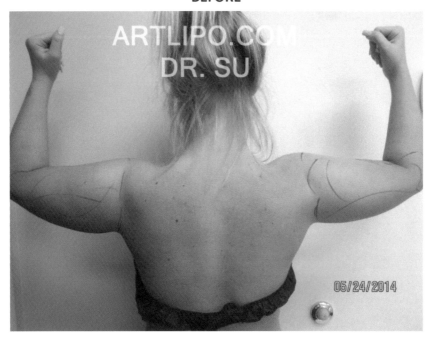

**AFTER**

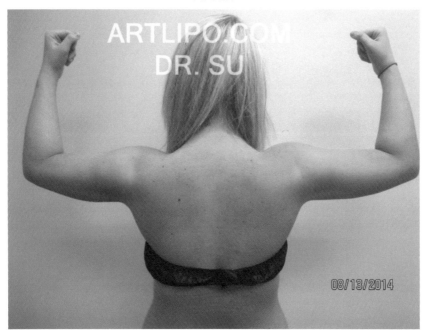

**Case 16** – A young college student with a petite-medium build, but a disproportionately large amount of fat on her arms since childhood. Her results were life changing.

**BEFORE**

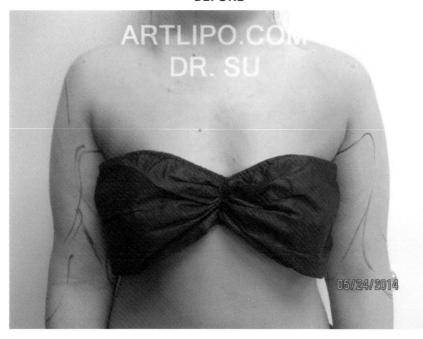

**AFTER**

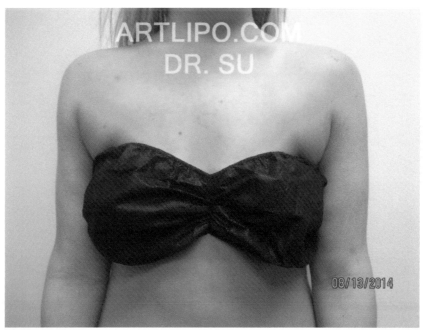

**Case 16** – continued. This view of the patient shows how much slimmer her whole body looks when the arms are slim. She even has slight shoulder definition.

**BEFORE**

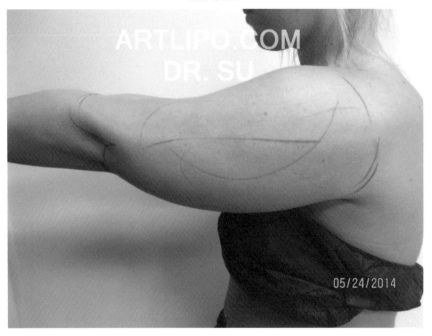

**AFTER**

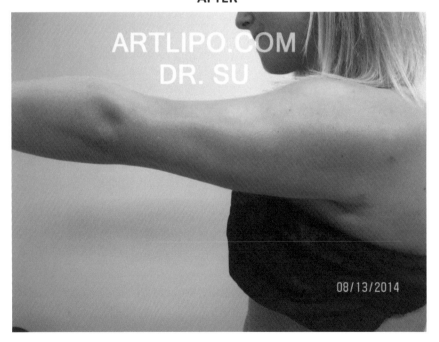

**Case 16** – continued. This side view shows the dramatic change in the size and shape of her arm.

# Group C

Patients with Moderate Fat Layer and Sagging Skin

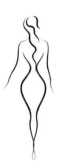

**BEFORE**

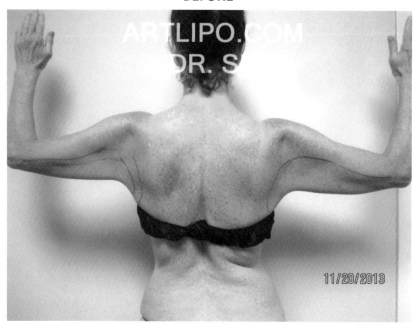

**AFTER**

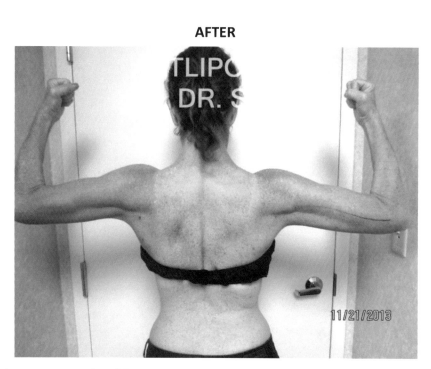

**Case 17** - This patient in her fifties had severely sagging skin—almost two inches hanging. Her fat was moderate and we expected possible skin wrinkling. However, her skin retracted beautifully by the next day with very few wrinkles. The after photo was taken the day after surgery!

**BEFORE**

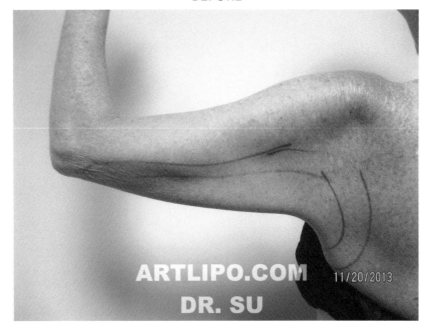

**AFTER**

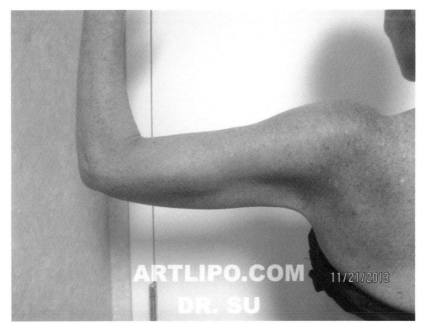

**Case 17** – continued

**BEFORE**

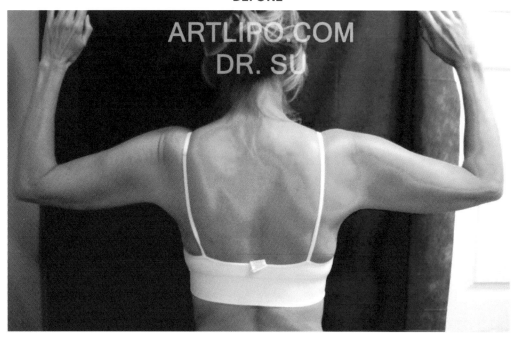

**AFTER**

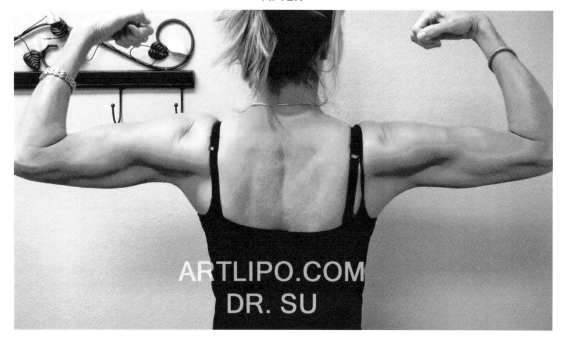

**Case 18** - This patient in her early forties had only moderate fat, but she had moderate skin sagging. It was surprising to see how well-defined her muscles were after her liposculpting.

**BEFORE**

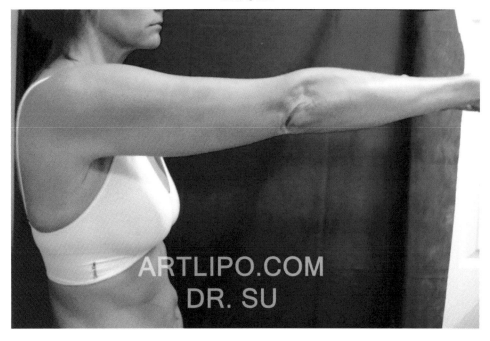

**AFTER**

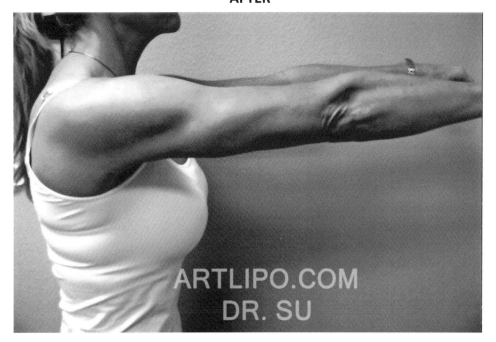

**Case 18** – continued

**BEFORE**

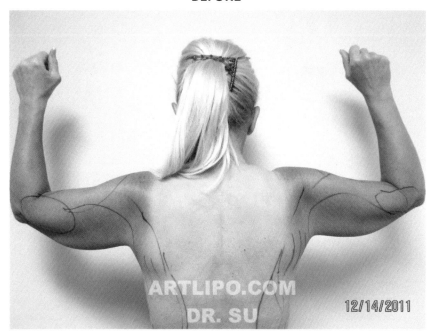

**AFTER**

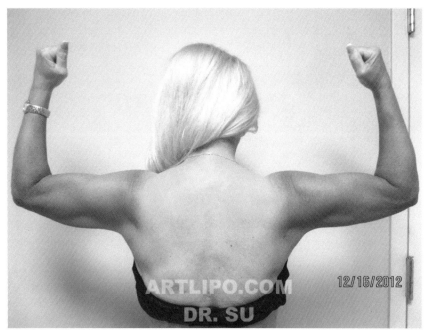

**Case 19** - This patient in her fifties had a large amount of fat and skin sagging. Surprisingly, she has great muscle definition and tone that was revealed after sculpting, and she has significant slimming without any skin looseness after liposculpting.

**BEFORE**

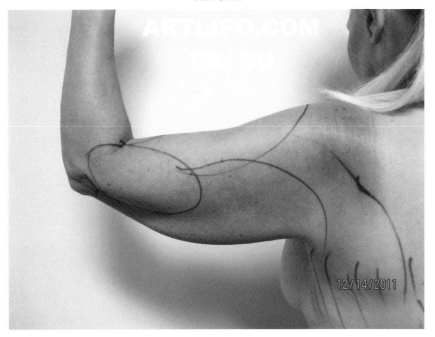

**AFTER**

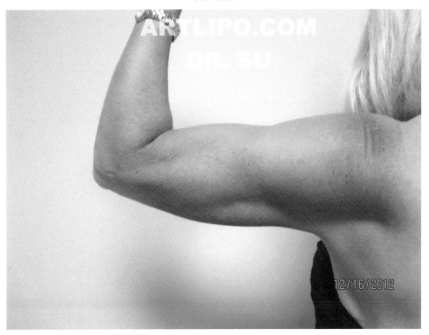

**Case 19** – continued

**BEFORE**

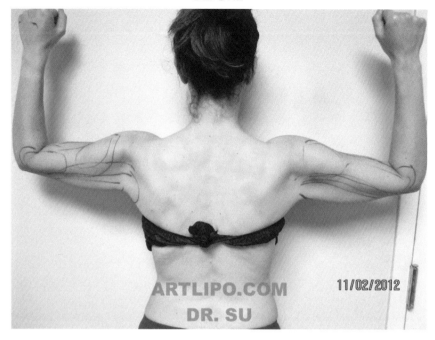

**AFTER**

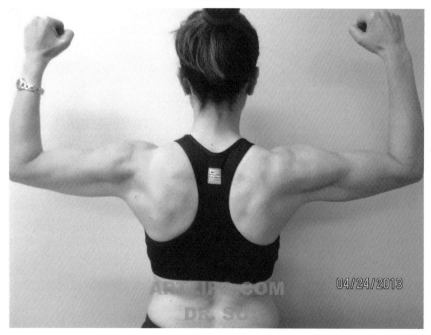

**Case 20** - This patient in her forties had moderate fat and moderate skin sagging. Her skin retracted very well, and the sculpting revealed some significant muscle tone.

**BEFORE**

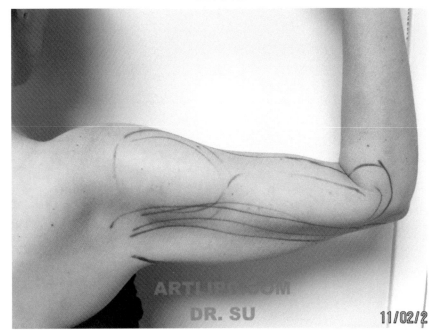

**AFTER**

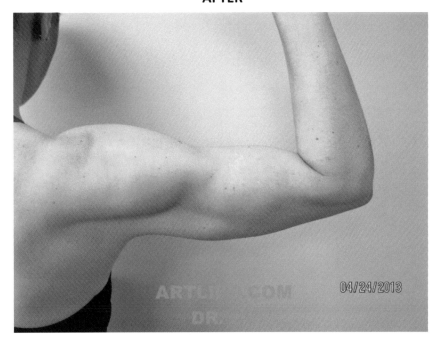

**Case 20** – continued

## Glossary of Medical Terms

—〰—

**abdominoplasty**  A cosmetic surgery procedure which removes excess skin and fat from the abdomen. Also called a *tummy tuck*.

**Aqualipo®**  A type of cosmetic surgery which uses water jets during the liposuction procedure.

**awake liposuction**  A type of liposuction surgery which is done without the use of general anesthesia.

**brachioplasty**  A type of cosmetic surgery which removes excess skin and fat from the upper arm . Also called an *arm lift* or *arm tuck*.

**cannula**  A surgical instrument used during liposuction. A cannula is a thin metal tube with holes along the sides near the tip. The diameter of the cannula can vary.

**connective tissue**  A type of body tissue that supports or binds other layers of body tissue. In layers of fat, connective tissue connects the skin with the muscle underlying the fat through tough, fibrous strands referred to as *connective fiber*.

**fat pad**  A mass of closely packed fat cells surrounded by connective tissue. Examples of fat pads are on the abdomen, buttocks, and thighs. Fat pads typically sag near the bottom (closest to the ground when a person stands) due to gravity.

**injectable therapy**  A cosmetic procedure which injects a substance under the skin to produce results that are usually not permanent. Also called *injectables*. For example, Botox®.

**Interactive Lipo Method**  A new method of awake liposuction created by Dr. Thomas Su.

**liposuction**  Cosmetic surgery which removes local areas of fat from the body using an instrument inserted under the skin and suction.

**medical spa**  A hybrid between a medical clinic and a day spa which offers cosmetic services such as injectables and laser therapy. Also called a *med spa*.

**SmartLipo™**  A type of cosmetic surgery which uses laser during the liposuction procedure.

**tumescent liposuction**  A type of liposuction where diluted local anesthetic is injected into the area that will undergo liposuction.

**VASERlipo®**  A type of cosmetic surgery which uses ultrasound during the liposuction procedure.

# Medical Disclaimer

The information is this book is intended only to provide a reader with a general medical information resource and to deepen the reader's knowledge of various liposuction techniques. None of the information included herein should be used as a substitute for a professional medical diagnosis or medical treatment.

Furthermore, none of the information in this book is intended to replace or be a substitute for any relationship that exists, or a substitute for any information, opinions, recommendations, advice, or counseling previously provided by any licensed medical, psychiatric, psychological, counseling, or social work professional.

Any reliance you place on such information from this book is therefore strictly at your own risk.

The author and the publisher both expressly disclaim all responsibility, and shall have no liability, for any damages, loss, injury, or liability whatsoever, including death, suffered as a result of your reliance on any information contained in this book.

This book also includes various before and after photographs of actual patients from the author's own liposuction clinic. However, no identifying information or Protected Health Information (PHI) is included for any patient photograph to actually identify the patient. Tattoos and other identifying marks were removed from some of the photographs to further protect the patient's identity. In addition, the author warrants all patients who have photographs included herein have signed a release form in their patient file and none of the photographs or text regarding these photographs provided by the author violate any provisions of the U.S. Health Insurance Portability and Accountability Act (HIPAA) of 1996 for protecting patient health information privacy.

In the event that any patient included in a photograph(s) herein objects at a later time to their use, the patient can contact the publisher in writing and clearly explain: (1) which photograph(s) the patient objects to; (2) how the patient knows the photograph(s) is one of him/her; and (3) formally requests removal of the photograph(s) from the book.

After consulting with the author, and if the information provided by the patient is actually valid, the publisher will remove any such pictures from new copies of this book as they are printed or generated.

# Model Disclaimer

This book includes a number of pictures of models that were licensed from their respective copyright holders. The licensed pictures include a model release and when appropriate, a product release.

These licensed pictures are subject to the disclaimers of their respective licenses and all of the disclaimers included herein.

The models in these photographs have been specifically selected to illustrate a desired natural toned and fit look.  None of the models has undergone any medical procedures provided by the author of this book.

This desired look may only be achieved on patients meeting specific criteria as determined by Dr. Su using the techniques described in this book.

The use of photographs of the models does not constitute or imply any endorsement, recommendation, favoring, or even any knowledge of any of the techniques described in this book, or the author, by the models.

The views and opinions of author expressed in this book also do not state or reflect those of any of the models in the photographs being used under purchased licenses.

Model-1  Veer Photo (OJP002072)

The person depicted in this photograph is a model and is being used for illustrative purposes only.

The model in the photograph does not use, personally endorse, or even have any knowledge of, any business, product, service, cause, association, medical technique, medical procedure, or other endeavor described in this book, or the author, of this book.

Model-2  iStock Photo/Getty Images (6217258)

The Content (photograph) is being used herein is for illustrative purposes only.  Any person depicted in the Content, is a model without any knowledge of anything described in this book, or the author, of this book.

# Trademark Disclaimer

This book includes the trademarks of others. These trademarks are used under the legal doctrine of *Nominative Fair Use*, by which a person may use the trademark of another as a reference to describe a product or service. The trademarks used herein were used under the legal doctrine of Nominative Fair Use because: (1) the product or service could not be readily identified by the author without using the trademark; (2) the author only uses as much of the mark as is necessary for the identification; (3) the author has done nothing to suggest sponsorship or endorsement by the trademark holder or any actual connection to the trademark holder; (4) the author has not used the mark in a disparaging manner; and (5) since the trademark use is only nominative fair use, it cannot and does not dilute the corresponding trademark in any way. However, if any trademark owner desires that their trademark be removed from this publication, please contact the publisher. The corresponding trademark will be immediately removed from all new copies of this book.

# Contact Artistic Lipo

If you would like to learn more about the Interactive Lipo Method or to a schedule a consultation, you can contact Dr. Su at Artistic Lipo.

## Artistic Lipo

6319 Memorial Highway

Tampa, Florida 33615

(813)886-9090

www.artlipo.com

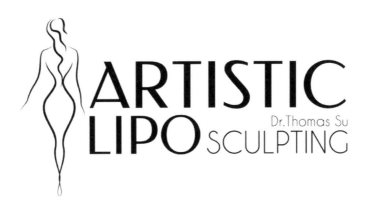

## About Coconut Avenue®, Inc.

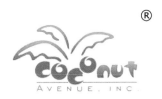

Coconut Avenue, Inc. is a publishing company founded by *Stephen Lesavich, Ph.D., J.D.* in 2007, in Chicago, Illinois. Dr. Lesavich, an award-winning author, is considered by many to be a self-help pioneer and visionary.

Coconut Avenue was founded on South LaSalle Street in the financial district, the heartbeat and pulse of the city of Chicago.

Coconut Avenue publishes books in a variety of genres, in most popular print and electronic formats. Coconut Avenue books are available worldwide in bookstores and on major e-booksellers on the Internet.

Visit Coconut Avenue online or on social media via links on:
coconutavenue.com

# An Award Winning Publishing Company

## Coconut Avenue®, Inc.

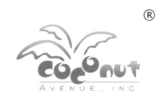

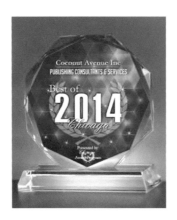

Coconut Avenue, Inc. was selected for the **2014 Best of Chicago Award** in the *Publishing Consultants & Services* category by the Chicago Award Program.

*"The Chicago Award Program recognizes companies that enhance the positive image of small business through exceptional service to their customers and their community. These award-winning companies help make the Chicago area a great place to live, work, and play."*

# Other Coconut Avenue® Titles

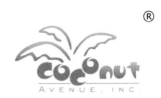

*Seven Letters That Saved My Life:*
*Seven Principles that Made it Happen*
Dottie Lessard

(Motivation, Self-Help)

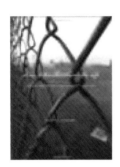

*The Plastic Effect: How Urban Legends Influence the*
*Use and Misuse of Credit Cards*
Polly A. Bauer and Stephen Lesavich, PhD, JD

**2013 Independent Publisher**
**Living Now Book Award**
**Gold Medal Winner**
**Judged Best New Book in**
**Finance/Budgeting Category**

**Amazon - Business & Money Books - Best Seller**

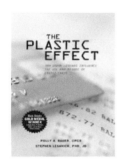

Coconut Avenue books are available worldwide in various print and electronic
formats in bookstores and on major e-booksellers on the Internet.

## Other Coconut Avenue® Products

FOR MORE INFORMATION ABOUT
OTHER COCONUT AVENUE®
AUTHORS, BOOKS, PRODUCTS, AND EVENTS,
PLEASE CONTACT:

**Coconut Avenue, Inc.**
39 S. LaSalle Street, Suite 325
Chicago, Illinois 60603 USA
(312) 419-9445 (v)
(312) 896-1539 (f)
email: info@coconutavenue.com
online: coconutavenue.com

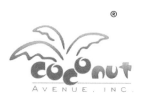

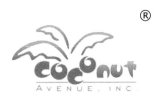

If you are interested in discussing the topics in this book on social media, please join us on Twitter at the hash tag **#CELEBRITYARMS** on ***@ArtisticLipo*** or ***@DoctorThomasSu***.

CPSIA information can be obtained at www.ICGtesting.com
Printed in the USA
BVIW12n0804190217
476582BV00012B/139